Leaving Life in the Fat Lane

Chris Catt, PsyD, HSPP, ACSM

Chicago Spectrum Press

4824 Brownsboro Center

Louisville, Kentucky 40207

502-899-1919

10 9 8 7 6 5 4 3 2 1

ISBN: 978-1-58374-248-8

DEDICATION

I dedicate this book to the loving memory of my mother, Thelma Joy Oetken. She's with God now, having worked tirelessly for Him while on Earth. She accepted me unconditionally and taught me how to live, love, and also to forgive. While her physical health failed her, her spiritual health was stronger than anyone I'd ever known. She was a true servant and she believed in the goodness of everyone, including me. Mom taught me to be kind, to be a good person and to love God. She left this world with some inspirational words: "From the city of gold, in a house built just for me, I'll be loving you, guiding you, and watching over you." I know she's been with me every step of the way.

I miss you Mom, and dedicate this book to you, a mother, a friend, and angel on Earth who is now in heaven. Thanks for the time you shared and for your inspiration.

PREFACE

There comes a time in your life's journey when you have to take a new road to get where you need to go. About twelve years ago, I had finished my doctorate in psychology and had a few years of practice under my belt. I decided to open a private practice and needed clients. I was initially licensed as Dr. Chris Oetken, but the name had always been a struggle for me.

Oetken is a German name and has a difficult German pronunciation. My family always pronounced it with an "E" as if the "O" were silent. Uncle Jim said the "O" was silent like the "P" in swimming. I know what you're thinking, but let's just say Uncle Jim is special. My clients looked for me under "E" and "A" in the phone book and on the directory in my office building lobby. Naturally this interfered with an otherwise good business plan.

I had talked to my 90-year-old grandmother Mary Oetken about the whole name dilemma some years before. She totally understood and blessed my decision to eventually change my name for professional reasons. Momo, as we called her, saw the practicality of the matter.

She thought like a young person and encouraged me in all of my life goals. We discussed the matter while eating cheese puffs and drinking a beer—she never drank more than half and it had to be the cheapest beer on the market. Momo was a great advisor and packed a lot of wisdom into that four and a half foot body. Still, in my eyes, she was always a giant. When she spoke, I listened. While flying to a conference in the south one year, I met a PR consultant to the Nashville stars. She said try to choose a name with a nice ring to it, where the first and last name start with the same sounds. After coming home from that conference, I met a person named Catt and he gave me permission to use the name. There was one other Catt in the local phonebook, so I called and told her I wanted to use the name, which she agreed to. I went to the courthouse and paid $28.50 for my new professional identity.

The Chris Catt name works well. My clients can find me, it has a nice ring to it, and it has been good for business. Sometimes change is necessary to move forward, but you don't have to forget the person you used to be either. I think Chris Catt is healthier, happier, and more successful than Chris Oetken was, but Chris Oetken, with the help of his family laid a good foundation.

I still remember that talk I had with my grandmother, and the encouragement she gave me to move ahead and take a different road. She was a wonderful person, and I'm sure she's a true asset in heaven. I hope you, too, have someone to help you move forward, particularly as it relates to your health and wellness, although you can do it with the name you already have. Save the $28.50 and use it to buy some healthy food.

ACKNOWLEDGMENTS

I always wanted to write a book but my ADHD, a short attention span, makes it challenging. I started the process in January of 2009 when I had a burst of post-holiday mania. I probably wrote two-thirds of it during that time, within just a few weeks. I wrote at 5:30 each morning. After that, there were numerous stops and starts. My second burst of creativity came at the Guatemalan orphanage I visited for the third time in January of 2010.

Health and wellness are passions of mine, plus my new healthy habits saved my life. I felt I had to share my story with others. I kept plodding along with revisions, re-writes, and adding new material. I wanted to keep it a simple read, information people could relate to, and also things that could be life changing like they were for me. I have to thank God for keeping me going. When I'd start to get discouraged, He gave me the thoughts I needed to forge ahead. That "still, small voice" can be pretty helpful if you just slow down enough to listen. Like any author, I have to acknowledge and thank others as well. My friend from St. Paul Church, Mark Johnson, a seasoned writer, was good enough to read the manuscript and also took the time to do some edits, which was totally unexpected. Mark also helped me see how the many chapters could be put together into an organized framework.

Olivia Schneider, a psychology major at Eastern Kentucky University, worked for my company during the summer of 2010. She diligently and efficiently made the necessary changes to the document. She's really bright and it's my understanding that she made straight A's in her last semester in school. She'll probably make a great psychologist.

Megan Resch and Myles Gann also helped out tremendously as student readers. Both of them attend Bellarmine University and are super bright seniors. They read the book from a student's perspective and offered suggestions as to how the book could be used to supplement existing wellness textbooks. I also want to thank Ann Rich, a good Christian friend, who works for a non-profit that records books for the blind. Ann was willing to volunteer her time as a reader.

She's a busy woman, keeping up with her husband Mark and two college-aged kids. Ann generously devoted her time doing a read through of the book and offered honest feedback for me to ponder.

My brother Todd was also helpful. He read through the book, offered nothing but positive praise and also contributed his own section on attitude. He read the initial manuscript in very rough form and then did a re-read with his girlfriend Sheila, while he was sidelined in the hospital for a few days. If I ever had a negative thought, I never shared it with Todd. He's all about the power of being positive.

My father Jerry Oetken was encouraging, as was his wife Phyllis. He always wanted to write a book himself but Parkinson's disease has taken away both his ability to write and to use a keyboard. He's been a real inspiration though in the way he's fought the disease for over nineteen years. His perseverance has been an inspiration to me and has kept me going even during times when I felt discouraged. He's never given up and I couldn't either.

Dorothy Kavka, at Evanston Publishing in Louisville, did a great job reading the manuscript and making editorial changes as needed. She has a great eye for the big picture. Her associate Sherry Welch was also an asset to the project. She was wonderful at explaining the overall publishing process and was patient with me along the way, as was their graphic artist, Will Peppers. If you ever want to self-publish a book, these folks are the best.

My daughter Sophia was helpful in making the changes Dorothy suggested. She spent three days, painstakingly making the changes that came from the publisher. This was a huge sacrifice for a 16-year-old because it interfered with texting, Facebook, and socializing in general. I think it interfered with her chores, too, but she wasn't much bothered by that. My wife Pia was somewhat reluctant, at first, to be involved in the project. She knows I have trouble with criticism and didn't want to hurt my feelings. While I asked for advice, I didn't always like it or take it. As the project progressed, she supported me in the endeavor and offered her thoughts and opinions whenever asked. Towards the end, she offered some editorial advice and was very supportive about my completing the project.

I can't conclude without thanking Heine Brothers Coffee. The good folks there were very understanding about the many hours I spent at the prime table at their Gardiner Lane store. The rent there was so reasonable. It was like having my own writer's lair in the corner and the bonus was, it was totally furnished. They let me use the plush leather chairs at no extra charge. If you're in Louisville, and want good coffee, go see them. You don't even have to be a writer.

FOREWORD

This book is organized into five main sections. I've grouped the chapters into sections clustering around specific themes. Please read on so you at least have a mental framework for what you'll be getting into during the course of your reading. Knowing what to expect helps you retain the information better.

In section I, I introduce the concept of wellness and discuss how many of us easily get off track with our health and habits. I was in the fat lane of life and was on the road to a premature death based upon my lifestyle. The insurance companies knew it even more than I did. My story is probably somewhat extreme but I share it anyway. I'll take you through one of my typical workdays. It's a good place to start and we all need to look at our lifestyles and daily patterns just to gain perspective.

Section II is about facing up to the truth and letting go of denial regarding your unhealthy habits. It deals with gathering information and laying the foundation for change. I also share a very inspirational story about my father and how a change in lifestyle saved his life. Exercise before being diagnosed has allowed him to live with Parkinson's disease for over nineteen years.

I'll talk about changing from the "outside in" throughout Section III. The changes I made are things you'll want to adopt as well. In this section, I'll tell how, you too, can do it. Additionally, I'll share some motivational stories and highlight the importance of setting goals.

Without short and long term goals, you'll drift like a ship without a rudder.

Section IV focuses on changes you'll want to make from the "inside out." There is so much evidence now that supports the mind/body connection. You'll learn how to adopt a more positive attitude and deal better with emotions. In this section, you'll also learn the importance of passion, laughter, and even quiet time.

In the final section, I'll take a look at a wellness versus a disease focus and the implications for healthcare in America. As a people, our lifespan is now going backwards. I'll encourage you to practice the methods I teach in this book and also ask that you share them with others. Lastly, I end with some motivational words and predict success for you along your journey.

E-reading & Interacting with the Book

The book is meant to be interactive in a way that makes you think about your patterns and gain awareness. I encourage you to write in the book where space is provided, to set goals, answer questions, and enlist accountability partners along the way. Feel free to highlight areas that you really need to work on and specific focus areas you may want to come back to later. Even though the book is designed to be an easy and practical read, I suggest you take your time as you work through it.

If you're doing e-reading, you're encouraged to take an interactive approach as well. Essentially, I've left your version in the originally paperback format as to not lose the workbook -like approach. It's important for you to write some things down and answer the questions as you move through the book. You'll also want to enlist accountability partners as needed, share your goals with them, and have them sign and witness your goals as you write them out. Accountability is a wonderful thing and believe me, it will keep you moving in the right direction. I suggest getting a journal to keep with you as you read. Use the journal as a companion to your e-book and simply respond to the questions as if you were writing in a hard copy. It truly helps to see your reflections in writing and by keeping it an active process, you'll be much more successful in the end.

Letter to Students

I appreciate you purchasing this book and reading it as part of your class assignment. The book tells how I damaged my health over the years, beginning when I was in college. While the book's primary audience is people your parents' age, the problem behaviors start at your age or even earlier. So often, you simply repeat the patterns you saw in your family. AA people say, "If you do what you've always done, you get what you've always gotten." This is true.

As you read this book, I want you to learn from my mistakes. The choices you make now will dramatically affect your health when you're twenty to twenty-five years older. Young people never think they'll age but believe me, it does happen. When you're a college graduate, a successful career person/professional, and enjoying good economic success, you don't want to be limited by ill health. Emotional well-being and good health really are priceless. In many cases, once they're damaged, you can't get them back regardless of how much money you have in the bank.

Flip to the Appendix in the back of the book and review the discussion questions before you launch into reading the book. This is important. You'll want to reflect on the questions and be able to answer them once you're done reading. Your professor will use the questions to facilitate in-class discussion about the book. This is most effective when the class is broken up into several small groups with each group having a facilitator.

I think you'll find the book both interesting and enlightening. You'll learn how to successfully make changes in your life and gain awareness about your physical, emotional, and spiritual aspects. A sincere effort to learn the concepts will help you protect your health for the future.

All the concepts will apply to your parents as well. Feel free to pass the book on to them. You'll be practicing the technique of "paying it forward."

I hope Leaving Life in the Fat Lane is a good read for you and I thank you in advance for the time you'll invest in it. Lastly, I wish you well and most of all I wish you wellness both now and in the future.

–Dr. Chris Catt, Psy.D. HSPP, ACSM

Contents

1. Leaving Life In the Fat Lane: An Overview of Chris Catt's Turning Point

I WAS A SUCCESSFUL and driven middle-aged psychologist when the insurance companies gave me the bad news. My self-inflicted schedule had me driving between multiple clinic locations and seeing twelve patients a day. Ironically, I was evaluating people who had trouble working, since a number of my patients didn't take care of themselves or their health. Some were simply broken down from the hard physical labor they had done over the years. The coal miners certainly fell into this category.

Evidence suggests that lifestyle choices probably account for 90 percent of health related problems. A smaller number, maybe ten percent of people with health issues, are victims of bad genes, environmental circumstances, random accidents, and bad luck. Some things you just can't control.

As a teen, I smoked a bit. Mainly, I smoked to be cool. I didn't smoke for the taste or to destroy lung tissue. I got over this vice quickly. My patients didn't get over it and nowadays it's not so cool. Smoking practically makes you an outcast, yet for lots of people, it remains their primary pastime. Especially unnerving are patients with asthma and emphysema, the ones who gasp for air, yet continue to smoke. Some people even carry portable oxygen tanks just to leave their homes, only to hook back up to the bigger tanks when they return. My own mother had this addiction as well. Her three-pack-a-day habit eventually killed her.

I was a health psychologist after all. I was college educated, smart, sensible, practical, and conservative. I considered myself well informed; I was a professional who should have known better. I generally did the right thing, didn't take risks, and was ultra responsible. In my mid 40s, I was denied both health insurance and life insurance because the insurance people considered me at risk for a premature death. I was uninsurable based upon the state of my health and my lifestyle. Things had to change. I needed to do more than talk about health. Taking control of my own health needed to become a priority for me.

After being denied both health insurance and life insurance, I had to wake up, see the truth, and look at myself as I really was. The hurried life, the hectic schedule, the fast lane I lived in had truly become the fat lane. I was on the road to a heart attack and didn't even know it. Those health insurance denials saved my life. I was 50 pounds overweight, had high cholesterol, didn't drink water, and avoided exercise. My eating schedule was unpredictable, and fruits and veggies were for people who had time for them. I ate most of my meals in my car while driving between my offices.

When the health insurance agent referred me to the state's high-risk pool for insurance, an alarm bell went off inside my head. I was being placed in the same category as people with cancer, lung disease, diabetes, and other chronic illnesses. The insurance company considered me a liability, a bad bet. I was on the wrong road. I was in the fat lane, and at this pace, I'd be meeting my maker sooner rather than later. I had to change course, not just for myself, but for my family as well.

A journey of a thousand miles starts with the first step. First you have to know where you are and how you got there before you can change course. I was able to look at my lifestyle, evaluate it, make changes, and get healthier. The good news is that you can do it too. In a year's time, you can change many of your unhealthy habits and be well on your way to a better quality of life, and in this book I'll tell you how to do it.

This book chronicles my journey from high-risk to high-health, and tracks the changes I made from reacting to responding. It tells my story and offers insights on how you, too, can change course and get out of the fat lane of life. While some people cheat fate, the fat lane generally leads to death, sometimes quickly and sometimes slowly. Yet you have the ability to get back on track and to make your health a priority. If you choose to change your habits a little at a time, your quality of life can be so much better, with more energy, more joy, better moods, and more mobility. I hope my story helps you choose health for you, your family, and your future.

A Day in the Life

You've heard the story about the lost cow that ended up several pastures from home, right? He didn't get there all at once. That cow strayed one clump of grass at a time. Eventually, he couldn't find his way back. People are like this, too, including me. Little by little, I strayed from a healthy lifestyle and moved towards the one that was killing me.

I'm a big fan of AA sayings because they really tell it like it is. I like the one that states, "If you do what you've always done, you'll get what you've always gotten." Another is, "the definition of insanity is doing the same thing and expecting a different result."

My daily lifestyle truly had become insane, and maybe yours has become crazy as well. I had strayed far enough that I needed to just stop and take notice. You, too, might also be at the point of needing some self-reflection and evaluation.

I'll describe one of my typical days for you, so you'll have a before and after perspective. Maybe you'll identify with some themes that are also occurring in your life, things that really need to get your attention before it's too late. I'm guessing you're not as far off track as I was.

Even so, we all have some unhealthy patterns that need adjusting.

****

The alarm rings at 5:00 AM. I bang it twice with my fist and bolt out of bed. I stumble into the shower, burn myself with hot water, and then get soap in my eyes. The morning's just begun and already, I'm irritated with life. Jumping out of the shower, I trip trying to put my pants on. Something about being tired makes your leg go in the wrong pant leg every time. More irritation!

In my rush to get going, I run out the door without patient files and car keys. I search for the spare key in the dark of a backyard shed, and of course there's never a light when you need one. Going back into the house, I grab my keys and my files. I then make one last bathroom stop, which my dad taught me to do as a child before any big car-trip. A quick look in the mirror shows that I've buttoned my shirt wrong and missed a large patch of whiskers on my face.

The human condition is difficult in the early morning. There are too many tasks to do just to face the day, too many things that need to be done before you're even truly awake. Sometimes you get by on autopilot mode, but more often you don't. Also, when it comes to morning glitches, there tends to be a domino effect. One wrong move leads to the next and so on. These are the mornings when you just can't wait to smell the coffee—it just happens to be a mile away.

I think about coffee long before I ever taste it. The pioneers used to make it in their kitchens but now that just takes too long. I glance at the coffee maker as I rush out the door, determined to reach the coffee house and plop down $2.29 for this black gold. The pioneers must have had more time to kill than this modern day psychologist. My car knows the way to my local Heine Brothers Coffee House in Louisville, KY. It gets me there every morning, although I'm rarely conscious of the journey. Other coffee pilgrims are already there to get their fix. I figure it's not really a problem unless you snort it or smoke it, and since I'm still content to drink it, I consider it one of the better legal addictions.

The coffee baristas are good. They know my thoughts. I don't even need to speak. The barista takes my travel cup and fills it. No words are necessary as they take my coffee card and swipe it. Black coffee tastes way too much like coffee so I stumble to the cream table. Choices…choices…skim, whole milk, or half and half—what will it be?

My cholesterol is dangerously low…so I think…I reach for the half and half. It's thick, tastes good, is loaded with fat, and dilutes the taste of straight coffee. Skim is a waste, since it tastes like white water. Whole milk is half way to half and half, so why bother? My arteries are too clear anyway…so I think. Mornings are hard for most of us and smelling the coffee seems to make it better. Only later, when more informed, would I come to appreciate the phrase "Wake up and smell the coffee," as it applied to my health and to my lifestyle.

Food on the Fly

Coffee in hand, I'm on the highway racing to work. While some work is local, today's clinic is a two hour drive. Naturally my gas gauge is on E. How does this happen? I'll have to make some hard choices: do I stop at the next gas place or risk getting to the one that's usually the cheapest in the state, the Flying J? I risk it, passing up a good price and hoping to make it to the lower price place without running dry. I make it, but the per gallon price is six cents more than the place I passed, plus I could have run out of gas. It's like being at the grocery where regardless of the line you choose, it's the slowest.

Once I have gas in my tank, it's time to fuel my body. The fastest food in the morning resides under the golden arches. I scan the horizon looking for a sign. Mickey D's feeds lots of hungry people in the morning, and they're everywhere. The bright yellow arches just suck you right in. My car swerves whenever I pass one. I can't see twelve patients without eating first. I pull into the next McDonald's and realize that I'm late to the party. The parking lot is jam packed. Everyone beat me to it. Maybe I should have skipped the coffee, or maybe I should have skipped the gas. What was I thinking?

The drive-through is out. At this point, it's a wait-through with at least ten cars in line. What a concept. You talk to a sign from the comfort of your car and somebody hands out food from a window. I opt to be more like a pioneer, park the car, and walk into the restaurant.

I dodge vehicles and almost sustain injury getting across the parking lot. People stare at me from their cars as if somehow I'm less evolved than they are. I'm physically going after my food and am willing to interact with the counter-people.

I make it in and get to the counter. Fast food is now slow food because the counter people are all focused on the drive-through people, and after all, they're the majority.

I ponder what to get from the pictures on a board. People used to read menus, but now they just look, point, and say a number. There are large fluffy biscuits filled with sausage, egg, and cheese. The hash browns look good too, and they're cooked to a golden brown color. Then there's the all too scrumptious biscuits and sausage gravy. All the choices are a cardiologist's nightmare.

A worker greets me. She speaks English, which is good since my Spanish is marginal. I settle on food I can cram in my mouth while driving, drinking coffee, and talking on my cell phone. Two sausage, egg, and cheese biscuits should go well with some hash browns and biscuits and gravy. I get in my car and position the food before driving. I open the breakfast biscuits and position them on the dash. I open the sausage gravy and place it in the second console cup holder next to my coffee. The biscuits, I open and place on the passenger seat for easy access. When you eat most meals while driving, it is important to position the food for maximum safety.

On the road again, I travel down the highway and calculate the safest speed at ten miles over the limit. This is what the authorities expect you to drive. Eleven miles over is simply wrong and is breaking the law. Going about 80, I grab the breakfast biscuit and cram half of it in my mouth. I chew vigorously and wash it down with coffee. I learned to drive with my knees to make it safer to drive while eating. Something has to stabilize the wheel while both my hands are in use. I gobble down both of the sandwiches. At this point, I've eaten my grains, my meat, and my dairy. Three food groups and 1000 calories down the hatch!

The next course is the biscuits and gravy. Briefly, I drive with both hands. All is well. My speed is steady at 80. Feeling safe once more, I put my knees to work steering the car, which is one advantage of having long legs. I work at finishing my breakfast holding the gravy cup in one hand and the biscuits in the other. Skillfully, I alternate between biting the biscuits and drinking the gravy. This maneuver isn't for amateurs. Timing is everything; one wrong move and you can either choke or end up with gravy in your crotch. After all, I was going to see patients and needed to look professional.

Finally, the McDonald's attack is over. I've covered some miles, filled my belly, and coated my arteries with a thickened gray-brown film. My stomach rumbles in protest, but I don't listen. Denial seems more convenient than doing things differently and change is hard!

The Rumble Seat

A little closer to the office but not close enough, it started. It's what I call the rumble. It's that point after eating grease that your stomach starts to talk to your brain. At first it's subtle and you try to ignore it hoping it goes away. Denial works for only so long. The sounds get louder, those intestinal sounds that say, "Something bad is going to happen." The rumbling becomes louder and more frequent. Denial is no longer an option. The moment of truth is near, and you have to admit you ate something that your stomach doesn't like.

Grease isn't a food group and early hunter-gatherer people didn't get much of it. Typically the diet was high fiber/low fat. Fruits, berries, roots, and occasional venison did the body good. Most tribal people ate food the body was meant to eat, and they had to exercise to get it. They walked about ten miles a day, which helped keep them lean and also aided digestion. All of this sounds good but doesn't help when you're "ready to rumble." There's a price to pay when you eat the wrong stuff. I had eaten from at least five food groups; grains, meat, dairy, caffeine, and grease.

There was a roadside gas station where I was able to get some relief. I exited quickly, tried to look innocent, and not be spotted. No time to linger, since I'm already late. Finally, back in the safety of my car, I soothe myself with more coffee. I need to hurry. I have to get down the road quickly. I need to go to the office and start seeing patients with multiple medical problems, people who eat the wrong stuff, people who don't manage their stress, and people with bad lifestyle habits. This is ironic isn't it?

In my quest to be successful, I was eating and hurrying myself to death. Finally at the office, I rumbled some more. I wasn't so different from the people I came to evaluate. Like some of my patients, I was making bad choices everyday and maintaining unhealthy habits.

It goes back to that AA slogan, "If you do what you've always done, you get what you've always gotten." How true…how true!

Caution—Men Working

Finally, I was now in my element; I was in the work zone. My patients awaited me. Usually, the first one was around 8:00 AM. I greeted John Doe cordially, made initial small talk and then proceeded with a psychiatric interview. Most of my patients have multiple medical problems along with some accompanying mood disorders, such as depression or anxiety. Mr. Doe was no different. Bad life-style choices had left him with heart disease, obesity, type II diabetes, peripheral neuropathy, high blood pressure, chronic back pain, gastroesophogeal reflux disease, and chronic fatigue. He hadn't taken care of himself along the way and now faced being disabled at age 49.

Body, mind, and spirit—they all go together. His mood was depressed, and he suffered generalized anxiety along with some panic anxiety when he couldn't breathe. Mr. Doe couldn't sleep at night due to financial worries and back pain. His body was broken as was his spirit. I sympathized with his plight and gathered all the needed information to complete the consultation. His story was not unlike my own. He ate a high fat/low fiber diet and drank cola instead of water. Exercise was not a priority for him. He worked too much at a stressful job and didn't take time to rest. He drank a lot of coffee and then self-medicated the anxiety with alcohol.

Obviously, his condition didn't develop overnight. Like the previously mentioned lost cow, Mr. Doe slowly and gradually strayed from his home pasture and got away from doing what was good for him. A cigarette after lunch and dinner led to a two pack a day habit. Morning coffee became a pot a day habit. For him, dessert after dinner led to ice cream before bed. A beer after work turned into beer while watching the news, during the ball game, and one before bed, which was to help him sleep.

During the early years of marriage, he and his wife ate dinner at the kitchen table. This evolved into couch dining, which unfortunately, has no cut-off time as long as the TV is on. Couch time and beer time replaced Mr. Doe and his wife's after-dinner walks. Since he had put on a lot of weight, the walks had become increasingly more difficult, while the couch was easy and comfortable. Mr. Doe had strayed from those things that were good for him. Unfortunately, getting lost is so much easier than finding your way back. I had to ask myself, "Am I all that different?"

My day continued. Patient one led to patient two, to three and so on. The morning moved towards noon and all of a sudden, I realized I had worked my way through lunch. I hadn't eaten since my early morning Mac attack. In the course of the day, I saw a total of twelve John and Jane Doe's, people with multiple medical problems, many of them self-inflicted, some not. In the midst of my busyness, I failed to drink water, but would periodically run next door to Hardees for more coffee. I was definitely dehydrated and over-caffeinated. My unhealthy habits were decreasing the quality of my days and the quality of my life.

Toward the end of the day, around 4 PM, my blood sugar crashed. My hands shook, and I felt irritated and weak as if I might pass out. I closed the office, hopped in my car, and sped to the local Thornton's quick mart for relief. I guzzled orange juice right out of the cooler case. I had to. The lottery ticket junkies were holding up the checkout line as usual. I'd seen the OJ thing work before with diabetic kids in a psychiatric hospital and it worked for me as well. I felt better and the shaking stopped. Being a well-educated man with a bit of common sense, I knew the cause was the lack of food. I needed food now.

Now, it was about survival. I knew I had to eat the first fast food I could find. There was no time to be picky. Ahead on the highway, I spotted my salvation in the letters KFC. The drive-through was jam packed with modern day road warriors; you know, people who no longer walked for their food.

I parked my car, walked into the restaurant and quickly scanned the picture menu. Original recipe drumsticks are always a good choice for eating while driving. I also chose the large mashed potatoes with extra gravy. There's some preparation involved in making my order into driving food. At the counter, I vigorously mix the potatoes and gravy with a plastic spoon and I add a little hot water to thin it out and make it drinkable. DUI of mashed potatoes and gravy is not illegal.

Relieved to have food in hand, I jump in my car and head for home. It had been a busy day, with lots of patients, reports to do, and no time to eat or drink. I got on the highway and reached my cruising speed of the speed limit +10. My survival instincts kicked in and my knees naturally took the wheel. I used one hand to move a drumstick to and from my mouth, while using the other hand to manipulate the gravy container. In this situation, the cadence of alternating hands is so very important. I would bite the chicken, and then drink the potatoes and gravy to help wash it down. All was well with the world. I was using both hands to eat, my knees to control the car, and my ears to listen to the radio news of the day. Eating at a table was way overrated, so I thought.

Having finished what I considered a task, I threw the chicken box on the floor of my car along with the bones. I detest littering, so I trash my car to protect the environment. After finishing the gravy, I threw it towards the passenger side floorboard and was skillful enough to hit the box. I felt relieved yet sick at the same time. The chicken grease had started to irritate my stomach, and I don't think my colon was far behind. In my effort to get home quickly, my mobile meal had added at least two additional emergency relief stops. In my hasty efforts to fuel my body, I had unconsciously repeated my morning pattern. Somewhat weakened by the whole ordeal, I would need more coffee to be alert, drive safely with my knees, and concentrate on cell phone calls all at the same time. None of this was easy.

Coffee to Go—Please

My trip home to Louisville would take about two hours. I needed coffee; yet good road coffee can be a bit elusive. In the city, quality caffeine is plentiful. Louisville, Kentucky is coffee house heaven, right after Seattle. Good coffee is harder to find when you're on the road. Gas station coffee is questionable at best. On my first attempt, I stopped at a place that had a pot of tepid warm and thick black liquid that used to be coffee. The creamer option was generic powder. It was definitely a pass.

I had a long drive ahead of me and I needed quality coffee to survive it. I exited a way down the road at a truck stop. The coffee smelled good enough, but the half and half curdled as it hit the coffee. Bummer… another failed attempt. I drove some more until I spotted a Circle K. From my experience I knew this was good coffee, and they even have the tasty French vanilla creamer, a flavored mix of chemicals that helps coat the arteries. I got the coffee, doctored it up, and was on the road again towards home. Just down the road on the interstate, I saw a sign for a new Starbuck's. My timing was always just a little bit off.

Finally, about a half hour from home, I had to make one final stop. This time it was a Thornton's. They're known for their good Dunkin' Donuts Coffee. It smelled great, so I loaded up with the 16-ouncer. I had to add the French vanilla half and half of course. Naturally, the Dunkin' Donuts Coffee and the Dunkin' Donuts go hand in hand, plus they're right next to each other. What else could I do?

I used a ratio of one donut per eight ounces of coffee, so I would definitely need two. Sour cream cake is the best kind, besides I thought the sour cream would help coat and protect my stomach from the caffeine. Plus, the donut covered two food groups…grain and dairy. Back on the road, I used the alternating hands, drive with the knees, speed limit +10 techniques once more. Surely this tried and true method would have me home in no time.

My journey was almost complete.

Home Sweet Home

I was finally home after a hard day's work. My nerves were shot from seeing lots of patients, the drive, too much caffeine, and, lastly, the city rush hour traffic. I needed some red wine to take the edge off. It's one of the first things I do after greeting my wife, my daughter, and the two cats. It immediately follows dumping all my paperwork, files, coins, pens, pencils, and other junk in the middle of the dining room table.

The wine is a cheap merlot from California uniquely bottled in a plastic skin and shoved inside of a box. I'm pretty sure the pioneers didn't have this invention either. Nonetheless, the wine serves its purpose, to take the edge off. One glass works well, so it stands to reason two might work better. The second is paired with the nice dinner my wife Pia prepared. She's a wonderful person to put up with me, and my unhealthy habits. I reasoned that the wine was for my health. It raises the HDL, the good cholesterol level, and also provides antioxidants to fight free radicals in the body. The other advantage of box wine is that you can't really see how much you're drinking. Sometimes ignorance is bliss (see Check Your Fluids / A NOTE ABOUT ALCOHOL).

After eating and kitchen cleanup, couch time seemed appropriate. I had been TV deprived and TV does provide a variety of human relationships that you can watch without having to participate. As I enter into my evening TV viewing trance, I can relax my mind a bit before worrying about the next day of work. The evening time on the couch then leads to nervous snacking and snacking out of boredom. At this point, I'm just forcing myself to eat peanuts, popcorn, cereal, string cheese, and even ice cream before bed. It's good to coat the arteries with fat so they stay supple during the night…yeah right!

Bedtime comes about 10 PM for me. My daughter Sophia goes to bed about 11. My wife might be up until a little later than me, too. She's addicted to shows such as House, Bones, and Without a Trace. TV addiction can be serious. The pioneers used to have to at least stand up, walk to the TV, and turn a knob each time they wanted to change the channel. They burned calories that way and channel surfing was virtually nonexistent.

Even though I go to bed early, my sleep isn't so good without a sleep aid. I use Trazadone, an older antidepressant that has the side effect of good sleep. I've put junk into my body during the day, failed to exercise, and used excess stimulants. My wife Pia says I snore and has diagnosed me with sleep apnea. Since her career was in TV news, I'm reluctant to accept her diagnosis. It's possible that I might snore, but a man has to be in denial about some things. I survived another day and sleep is always welcome if I can get it.

You can see that this health psychologist's day was not all that healthy. I had really bad habits and problematic patterns that I had repeated over and over for years. I needed one of those ah-ha moments. Maybe you've had these. Something comes over you like a light bulb going off in your head and you start to see things as they really are. Mine came with the help of the health insurance company and the life insurance company. I guess I needed to see the truth in black and white. I'll tell you how they helped me see the light and how you too can gain more awareness about your current health. Maybe your moment will come from reading this book. I hope it does. We can all do better for ourselves and for our families.

Use the space below to reflect on your own patterns. What habits do you have that are problematic? List the things you are doing that take away from your health and wellness. Right down what you think you're doing right as well. Self-reflection is the best place to start. Without it, change isn't possible. Please take time here to reflect and write in the book. This is meant to be an interactive self-help process and rushing through it won't help you.

____

____

____

____

____

Now in the space below, draw a picture of how you see yourself now and what you'd like to look like a year from now (your ideal shape / self). Don't be afraid to mark in the book. Make sure to put a date next to the second picture to give yourself a goal to strive towards.

2. KNOW YOUR NUMBERS

DECIDING TO IMPROVE your health is great, but first you have to know your numbers. Knowing your numbers is important. It gives you a place to start. You should know your BMI, which is the ratio of your weight to your height. There's a formula:

$$\text{BMI} = \frac{\text{weight in lbs.}}{\text{height x height (inches)}} \times 703$$

The normal range is 18.5 to 24.9 and is the range you want to get to. The 25 to 29.9 range is overweight and 30 and above is obese. When I got the wake up call, I was borderline obese. Maybe you're there too, or worse. Don't worry; it can change. It's just a place to start.

Waist circumference is a measurement used along with BMI at times. Android fat is the type that accumulates around the mid-section and results in visceral fat pressuring the internal organs. Waist circumferences of 35+ for women and 40+ for men increase the risk factors for heart disease and a number of other disease processes. Decide upon a healthy waist measurement for yourself. Maybe it's one you had when you were younger. Make it a goal to regain that waistline you once had.

Your lipid profile is also important. A total cholesterol number isn't all that helpful although the current recommendation is < 200 mg/dL. You also need to know the LDL (bad cholesterol number), the HDL (good cholesterol number), your triglyceride number and the overall ratio (Total Cholesterol/HDL). Your LDL should be < 100 mg/dL and HDL is heart protective at 60+ mg/dL. Your triglycerides account for 95 percent of fat stored in the body and should be < 150 mg/dL. An overall ratio (Total Cholesterol/HDL) of equal to or less than 3.5 is what you want. Lower is even better. It means that you've got enough good cholesterol to help ream out your arteries, keeping them clear while limiting the bad cholesterol that causes blocked arteries and heart attacks. Hospitals, health-care organizations, and health departments will often do these screenings at a very nominal charge. Some doc-in-a-box clinics offer these screenings, and local hospitals periodically offer them in grocery stores.

Your resting heart rate number is good to know. It's your heart rate when you first wake up in the morning literally before you start moving around. It's a measure of cardiovascular fitness. Practice finding your pulse on your wrist. Use any timepiece that measures seconds, and count your pulse for ten seconds, then multiply by six. Ideally, you'd like your heart rate to be in the 60s. Lower is better. If you're really out of shape, yours might be in the 80s. Don't panic. It's just a number and a place to start. It can all get better. I've managed to get mine to the low 50's over the past few years.

Body fat percentage is critical since excess body fat increases your risk for multiple diseases. A body fat scale will suffice if you don't have access to this service through your gym or your doctor. You simply have to do the measurement under the same conditions each time. The time of day needs to be the same, and your level of hydration needs to be consistent. Your water intake, and that time of the month for women, can affect the measurement. If you're reading this book, your number could be in the mid to high 30s. Don't despair because it's really just information. Ten to 25 percent is the recommended range for men while 18 to 30 percent is recommended for women. If you get it into the teens then you're practically an athlete. Just remember that for a woman, a higher fat percentage is expected. It has to do with reproduction and the survival of the species.

Blood pressure is a measure of cardiovascular health, too. 120/80 is good. Lower is better. High blood pressure is classified as 140/90. Your blood pressure is important to maintain. Excess pressure puts stress on blood vessel walls, increasing your risk of heart attack and stroke. High pressure can break plaque off of the vessel walls, sending a blockage to your heart. High blood pressure plus plaque build-up in the carotid arteries can lead to a stroke. The plaque breaks from the artery wall and causes a blockage of blood to the brain. High blood pressure is also the culprit behind aneurisms. The excess pressure can affect a weak part of the artery wall, resulting in a bulge and sometimes a rupture. Check your blood pressure either at home or at your local drug store or grocery store. Don't let the numbers freak you out. Just know that they could be lower.

Eventually, you want to have good numbers. These are achievable over time. A proper high fiber/low fat diet, regular exercise, portion control, and healthy habits will move you towards your goal. Your numbers are your baseline. They're just the starting line. The race you'll be running is a marathon, not a 40-yard dash. It will become a lifestyle and a process.

Check your numbers and write them down. Then make some changes, and don't check your numbers for a while. Getting out of the fat lane takes time. The important thing is that you start the journey. It will be worth it for you, your family, and even for your employer. It's hard to put a price on good health. Since poor health negatively impacts almost all areas of your life, good health practices really are priceless. Sounds like a credit card commercial doesn't it?

Within the next week, make a good faith effort to know your numbers and list them below. The second column is for recording the improved numbers you'll have six months from now.

	Today's Date	Six Months
BMI		
Cholesterol Ratio		
Resting Heart Rate		
Percent Body Fat		
BP		
Weight		
Waist Size		

Knowing your numbers should get your attention and motivate you to change. Once you know your numbers, you can start seeing the truth about your situation and go about taking the next step.

The Truth Hurts

There's something unsettling about applying for health insurance and filling out all of the required forms. You have to honestly answer questions about your health history and your health habits. It makes you sit up and take notice. They ask questions like, how many hours of exercise you perform per week, your alcohol intake, and questions about eating fruits and vegetables and other preventative practices. The weight question's a tough one, too. It's hard to write the number down. The question about waist size is equally unsettling.

I was no Jared of Subway sandwich fame, but I had encountered the middle age spread. My belly was blocking my view of the bathroom scale. I had added seven inches to my waist size. My 41" waist size put me at increased risk of multiple diseases. I had gained 50 pounds over the years, finally weighing in at 250 lbs. When you're 6'4" tall, it spreads out a bit, but it still shows in your face and in the tightness of your clothes. It's not healthy, and the insurance companies know it.

It's funny about insurance folks. They just don't want to take your word for things. Whatever happened to the trust-me mentality? At my convenience, they wanted to send someone to my office to take some blood, weigh me, and measure my waist, etc. My BMI of 28 put me in the overweight/obese category, and my cholesterol was around 250 (not good). I was denied both life insurance and health insurance since I was at-risk of developing numerous health issues. I wasn't a good bet for them to insure and I was considered a real liability.

The insurance people referred me to the state's high-risk pool, the pool for people with cancer and pre-existing conditions who couldn't get coverage. The premiums were astronomical and I simply couldn't pay them. I couldn't afford to get sick and couldn't even afford to die without life insurance.

It finally occurred to me that I would have to change, not just a token change, but rather a change that would be enduring. My life and my financial health depended on it. As much as I hated it, I resigned myself to change my lifestyle just a little bit at a time. Change that endures is more gradual than drastic. I did it, and you can do it as well. I'll tell you how. It all starts with awareness of where you are now regarding your health and habits.

Change Does a Body Good

Now I knew my numbers. I also knew they weren't good. I needed to lose about 50 pounds, drop my cholesterol about 70 points, take seven inches off my waist, and lower my blood pressure. I needed to make these changes while also working, seeing lots of patients, and managing my stress. My caffeine intake would need to decrease, and I would have to cut back on the alcohol as well. It was a lot to think about. The insurance people had already thought about it though. They knew the numbers and decided I was a bad bet for them. I was "high risk" in my current condition. I needed to change my ways.

My mom lives with God now but she had a great approach to life. She raised seven kids and didn't get overwhelmed. I went to her for advice one time when I was really stressed and overwhelmed with work, grad school, and my first marriage. "Chris," she said, "life is like a patio."

"Really," I thought, "like a patio."

She had a huge concrete patio right outside her back door. It was divided into 24 four-foot squares and the limbs of a giant walnut tree hung above it. Constantly, that tree dropped leaves, sticks, and walnuts onto that huge patio. The mess was overwhelming, and it was year round.

Mom's patio approach was the same way she approached life. She focused on one square at a time. She'd sweep up one square and pick up the debris. Following that, she'd move to the next square and so on and so forth. The process of sweeping just one square was her focus and not the end result. This kept her from freaking out about the size of the task. She encouraged me to do the same. "Break it down," she said. "Choose one thing and make the change. Get a small success and move to the next thing. It makes it more manageable."

I encourage you to take the same approach with your health. Use the "patio approach." It really works. Choose a place to start, one little square of the leaf covered patio. Decide to clean up that part of your life by making better choices. Start small, but make sure to start. You've heard that a journey of a thousand miles starts with the first step. Choose that step, a start date, and go forward. Maybe it's a walk after dinner, whole milk rather than half and half in your coffee, or grilled versus fried food. Substitute pretzels for potato chips, skip the third glass of wine, or buy turkey bacon instead of the real thing. Choose something that's doable, and plan to succeed. Just take the first step. After all, life is like a patio; start with the first square.

Just Do It

There's something liberating about that "ah ha" moment when you know you need to take action. You've decided. You're "the decider." It sounds almost presidential, doesn't it? It feels good to choose a goal and commit yourself to the process of change. You know your health can improve and the future can be better for you and for your family.

I'd experienced the moment and was ready to change. I knew I wanted out of the fat lane of life. I was determined to choose health and to start in the smallest of ways. I always heard that breakfast is the most important meal of the day. Why not start there, I thought. My typical breakfast involved the Mac attack as I cruised down the road. Biscuits and gravy, bacon, egg and cheese biscuits, and hash browns would have to go. I'd also need to eliminate those sour cream cake donuts that I loved.

I saw a movie once called, *What About Bob* that focused on "baby steps." I always remembered that concept. I needed a baby step while still preserving some old habits. I could change my breakfast food and yet still eat in my car while driving. I'd make a whole-wheat, peanut butter and banana sandwich before leaving for work in the morning. This breakfast had three food groups: grains, protein, and fruit. I never had fruit in the morning before, but was confident that I could adjust to it.

The morning sandwich making became part of my ritual. I took the whole wheat bread from the freezer and put it into the toaster. While toasting, I got out the tin foil and placed it on the kitchen counter. While the bread was still toasting, I peeled and sliced the banana in half and then lengthwise. Pop, up came the toast. I've already opened the peanut butter and skillfully spread the peanut butter in two swift strokes. I artfully arrange the four banana pieces on the bread like a puzzle and smash it altogether. The sandwich then gets wrapped in the foil and crammed into my coat pocket. I was now ready to roll and no longer ready to rumble.

In my car, cruising to work, I stopped at my favorite coffee house to get my morning fix. At least for now, I'd keep using the half and half, although I walked for it this time. I parked my car across the lot and hoofed it into the store. Surely, I burned more calories than just using the drive-through method. Back in the car, I smelled the coffee first then I took that precious first sip of the morning. Satisfaction! Not wanting to change too much at once, I eased onto the road and unwrapped my healthy breakfast sandwich. I savored every bite with the comforting knowledge that it was actually good for me.

My other bad habits remained. I still held coffee in one hand, the sandwich in another and drove with my knees. However, I felt good knowing that I made a small change that morning and one that I could continue. Several years later, I still eat the whole wheat, peanut butter and banana sandwich every morning. Over time, I've added other healthy changes to my routine. The first one though, is very important. It has to be one that will make a difference and also a habit that you can sustain.

Before reading on, reflect on the first change that you can make to move yourself towards a healthier life-style. You have to start at square one.

SQUARE ONE

Write the first change you plan to make as a start towards improving your health and wellness. Keep it simple and make it something that will give you an early success.

____

____

____

____

Graze Your Way through the Day

It occurred to me that hunter-gatherer societies probably ate throughout the day, as they would find food. Walk a bit, and then eat some berries. Walk some more, and then eat some nuts. A ways down the trail, eat some roots. Occasionally, they would eat lean meat, such as venison. The point is that large amounts of food weren't available at three prescribed times during the day. They ate less, and they ate more frequently than I did. A lot of their food was fiber, and it was nutritious.

I planned to become a grazer. In the morning I resigned myself to packing a grazing bag. I used a quart-sized zip-lock bag, so I could see what I had left throughout the day. Each morning I filled the bag with things I considered to be good for me. The key was variety and quality. The bag was declared a junk-free zone. I filled the bag with raisins, peanuts, V-8 juice, Crystal-Lite packets, bananas, string cheese, yogurt, apples, whole-wheat bagels, and so forth.

Over time, my daily eating habits changed. In the morning, I had my standard whole-wheat, peanut butter and banana sandwich. After that, I was a grazer. At regular intervals, I reached into my grazing bag and ate something. It had protein, veggies, fruit, dairy, and grains in it. I was now eating seven times throughout my workday. My body and my mind did better with my new habit. The peaks and valleys with my blood sugar were eliminated. I never shook from lack of food. My mind was focused on my work rather than survival. My nervousness decreased. I was merging out of the fat lane with no more fast food. I didn't need it. I was now a hunter-gatherer.

Move It More

Even with the right fuel, vehicles still need to move. Your body is a vehicle, and it's meant to move a lot. Think of your hunter-gatherer ancestors. They moved frequently. When hunting, food rarely would just walk up to them. They had to hunt, often traveling long distances. When they gathered, they did the same. Exercise was automatic for them. If they didn't walk five or ten miles a day, they didn't survive.

Times sure have changed. The distance from my den to my fridge is about twelve feet, which doesn't burn many calories. Your early ancestors may have died from extreme weather or famine, but I doubt they died of heart disease.

Just eating right wasn't good enough for me. I'd have to move more. Start small, I thought and don't fight for the best parking space. That is why I'd try to park farthest away from my office or take the farthest spot from the entrance to a store. A little forced effort would be good for me. I got a cheap pedometer and began tracking my steps. In the first week of my effort, I just tried to get a base-line count. I averaged about 2600 steps a day, or about a mile and a quarter. This included all walking around the house, walking done at work, and anything in between. Essentially, it started from the time I got out of bed until the time I went to bed.

In the second week, I decided to do better. I added some exercise walks, like two loops around the city zoo, walks to my favorite coffee house, and walks through the Highlands corridor in Louisville. This got my daily average up to around 6500 steps. I felt encouraged. My daily steps were now over three miles. To make my goal of 10,000 steps per day, I just needed to add some gym time. I got on the elliptical trainer for 30 to 40 minutes a day.

I was now getting at least 10,000 steps per day or about five miles. I continued monitoring this for several weeks using my pedometer. Most times, I was well over what I needed. Once my routine was established, I eliminated the pedometer. It takes several weeks to establish a new habit and if you're stubborn, it takes longer.

I started losing about one and a half pounds a week. I felt much better. My pants started to get big. I remember how excited I got when I was able to go down one hole on my belt. My new habits were working well. The extra activity made me feel better and I slept better! When I occasionally treated myself with ice cream, I felt less guilty. Within a year, I had shed about 50 pounds and I lost about seven inches from my waist. I had to buy new pants.

I was walking distances walked by my hunter-gatherer ancestors. My blood pressure came own, as did my heart rate. I was able to get health insurance and life insurance. Now, this was real progress. My BMI was now 23…just perfect. My body fat averaged around nineteen percent. I was in the best shape of my life in my mid-forties and I never thought it was possible.

You can do it, too, but you've got to get moving. Get the cheap pedometer, and do the same thing I did. Start with a baseline number for week one.

Just count your average steps per day with what you already do. Don't change anything at first. In week two, try to add steps. Then vary your routine and add exercise walks. Fight for the furthest parking space. Take the stairs instead of the elevator. Resign yourself to adding more steps each week until you reach 10,000 per day. At that point, you're walking five miles. You're practically a hunter-gatherer. You'll start feeling better. You've increased your calorie burn, so you'll start losing weight. Don't be discouraged. Healthy weight loss is between a pound to a pound and a half a week. Fast weight loss is the kind that doesn't last. In this case, slower is better.

You really want your lifestyle changes to be sustainable. Otherwise, you'll simply become another one of the million yo-yo dieters. You've started healthy habits, and you want them to last a lifetime. Fad diets don't work. Diet contests don't work. Only healthy habits work, and you can keep doing them forever.

You might have an occasional relapse. That's OK. Don't get back in the fat lane. At this point you're well on your way to good health. You're practicing prevention. You're preserving your health for the future. You're doing it, not just for yourself, but also for your family. You'll live longer, and you'll have fewer problems. You'll be happier with yourself, maybe happier than you've ever been. It's all worth it. You will succeed.

Old Habits Die Hard

Making changes in your lifestyle and maintaining the changes can be difficult. When I changed my unhealthy habits, I assumed it might be temporary. I hoped they would be permanent, but that's rarely the case with people. Enthusiastic attempts at weight loss are often short-lived.

A few years ago, a number of my family members started a weight loss contest. It sounded good in theory. They'd weigh in on New Year's Day and then try to lose as much weight as possible over the next ten weeks. Each of them would use their own weight loss, exercise, and diet strategies. The entry fee was $100 per person with winner getting a cash prize.

As you could imagine, $1600 is a lot of motivation and my family was very serious about it. That's a bunch of loot and each of them was determined to win it: brothers, sisters, cousins, stepbrothers, and stepsisters. They would all start out fast like Kentucky thoroughbreds coming out of the gate. Each would work hard, running towards the finish line. In the end, there would indeed be "the biggest loser" and "the biggest winner" at the same time.

My fabulous niece Amy was with the Fit-Kids Family Wellness program at the time and coordinated the effort. She's a motivational machine, a real dynamo and an expert on wellness. She gets her positive attitude from my brother Todd Oetken. Amy sent out encouraging e-mails, healthy recipe tips, and was the all around cheerleader. She wanted everyone to succeed and Amy knew, in the end, they'd all be winners. Periodically, Amy would have a weigh-in to see how people were doing. She encouraged everyone each step of the way.

Towards the end, the final weigh-in was scheduled. They were all sprinting towards the finish. The biggest loser was getting closer and closer to the prize. The prize was big so the loss would need to be big as well, and it was huge. Chris K. was the big winner. He ended up $1600 richer and 42 pounds lighter. He worked hard for it, took it very seriously, and took home the prize. Hopefully, he was healthier as the result. My cousin Mike lost a lot of weight, too. I think he came in second. There just wasn't any cash reward for second place. Mike's used to second place since I beat him every year with my holiday house decorating. He's a good cousin though.

Months passed by after the contest and the contestants gravitated back to their old ways. Their belts got tighter again, they relapsed to their old eating habits, and the rush to exercise subsided. People tend to gravitate back towards what they're used to doing. Real and lasting change takes sustained and ongoing effort before new habits are established. To get healthier, you have to do those things you haven't always done, and you have to force it long enough for new habits to take hold. Ten weeks is a drop in the bucket when trying to maintain healthy habits that will last a lifetime.

A year went by and most of my family were back in the same boat. Not all, however; a select few actually turned the corner. Come Christmas, the participants were all abuzz about re-instituting the contest. They talked it over while feasting on holiday foods and celebrating the birth of Christ. They talked some more, and then they ate some pie. After sampling the pecan pie, the pumpkin pie, and Aunt

Joan's killer brownies, there was a general loss of interest. Old habits die hard.

Fat Dads Finish Last

When I was a child, my dad was the picture of death waiting to happen. He was supposed to weigh 160, based upon his height of 6 feet tall. He weighed more like 220 or 230. His belly dun-lapped over his belt, so he couldn't even see the scale. He was overweight and was addicted to alcohol. My dad, Jerry Oetken, drank beer every night after work with my uncle, from five o'clock on at the local beer hall. Eventually, they came home drunk to answer to their angry wives. My brothers, sisters, and I were usually in bed by then. The men ate tavern cheeseburgers and fries to help soak up alcohol and sober them up a bit for the drive home. Rarely did they drive NUI (not under the influence). The grim reaper was knocking at my dad's door.

Dad's main exercise was the 12-ounce curls of a beer can. He was good at it, but with any repetitive motion you risk carpel tunnel syndrome. He and my uncle could polish off a case or two of beer a day. In addition, they ate fried chicken, fried chicken livers, and fried fish. Fruits and veggies weren't part of the picture. As a child, I got my exercise running for more beer for them. Dad didn't drink much water in those days, and during the work-week he drank coffee all day long. He developed high blood pressure, racing heart rate, and arrhythmias. His cholesterol was off the charts, and he was smoking cigarettes, cigars, and pipes. He was moving towards death's door.

Dad had an epiphany one day and realized he would die if he continued this behavior. He decided that he would change. We lived near a high school football field. He started out simply trying to walk from one goal post to another and couldn't do it. He became winded and stopped. The next day though, he'd try again. Determined, he kept at it. It got to where he could walk back and forth between the goal posts several times each evening. He eventually moved to the high school's running track and gradually started jogging. Initially he jogged 18-minute miles, a little faster than walking.

Dad persevered. He intended to change his habits and to improve his health. He gave up smoking, which was a huge step, and this improved his jogging exponentially. Eventually, he entered a 5K race and finished last for his age group. Undeterred, he kept training, and was feeling better and getting faster. A few races later, he moved up to a 10K, doubling the distance. He didn't finish last. He made progress. Eventually he became a runner and became faster and faster. Eighteen-minute miles became 14-minute miles. He eventually improved to running 8-minute miles and later 6-minute miles. A year or so into his transformation, he was winning races in his age group. Dad gathered a collection of medals, trophies, and t-shirts from all of his runs. He was eating right, had reduced his drinking, and was in the best shape of his life.

He started a running club before running was even cool—the Cherokee Road Runners, they called themselves. They logged lots of miles in our local Cherokee Park. He ended up running with the good runners in our town: names like Swag Hartel, Ken Combs, Alan Melcher, and so forth. Eventually he would run the Kentucky Derby Mini-Marathon and then graduated to marathon running. He became addicted to feeling good and started traveling to race marathons. One year he ran the Boston Marathon. He was in his mid forties at the time. Dad even ran an ultra-marathon once, covering 50 miles from Frankfort to Louisville, KY. He was no longer near death's door. He had transformed himself into a competitive runner, a vegetarian, and the picture of health.

In his 50s, Dad was running and noticed his foot dragging. He started dropping things. Handwriting became difficult. He tried to keep exercising for some years, but in his mid-fifties he was diagnosed with Parkinson's disease. He tried to run as long as he could but started having balance problems. It's a terrible diagnosis and most Parkies go downhill pretty quickly. My dad was a fighter, though. He'd see multiple doctors, take boatloads of medicine, and see some more doctors. He'd fight the disease with the determination of a world-class marathon runner. He quit running but kept exercising on an Airdyne and with dumbbells. His disease would be a marathon. Dad's 75 as this book goes to print and has had the disease over 19 years.

Attitude and determination can carry you through the hard times of life. He was no quitter. He kept his body active, and he kept his mind active. He read all about what he would face and talked to others about it. Dad went to support groups and he talked at support groups. Dad engaged himself in spiritual reading and also in a men's study group that eventually admitted women, a very progressive move. He continued to follow domestic and world news, manage his investments, engage in intellectual conversation, and he continued to drive a car until recently. The doctors said that his running probably saved his life. He was in great shape when he contracted the disease, and he continued his healthy habits even after the diagnosis.

In his seventies, his mind remains sharp. He walks daily on a treadmill and lifts weights. He'll have some occasional falls, a broken bone here or there, but is remarkably healthy, except for the

Parkinson's. In fact, he was in such good shape that, a couple of years ago, he became the first Parkie in Louisville to have a deep brain implant surgery. My dad responded well to the intervention and spoke on numerous panels and symposiums as the result. He also talks to patients considering the procedure and with patients recently diagnosed with Parkinson's. His pre-diagnosis exercise and his continued exercise have been his salvation. He is active everyday and he lives independently with his wonderful wife, Phyllis, and has no special in-home care. If he had remained a fat dad he would have finished last in this race. He was saved by exercise. Consider exercise good preventative medicine, and no, it doesn't have to involve marathons.

I'm proud of my dad and the changes he made in his life. If you're a fat-dad or a fat-mom, you can change too. Do it for yourself, your family, and for your children. Start your healthy habits today, even if you start small. Make the decision and the commitment. Set a goal for week one, even if it's just walking the length of a football field. You have to start where you are and progress to where you want to be. Baby step after baby step, my dad changed the course of his life. Without the change he would be dead right now from heart disease, emphysema, liver damage, or Parkinson's disease. Don't wait. Choose to change. Remember my favorite AA slogan, "If you do what you've always done, you get what you've always gotten." You've got to get out of the fat lane to start.

Check Your Fluids

In the fat lane of life, you tend to neglect your vehicle. Not only do you put in the wrong fuel, but you neglect your other fluids as well. Fluids are important for both vehicles and bodies. They lubricate parts, deliver fuel, carry oxygen, and help eliminate waste. To be healthy and to get out of the fat lane, you need the right fluids.

I used to think we just needed enough liquid to get through the day; about 64 ounces. That was wrong. Not all liquids are created equal. My 64 ounces was always in the form of coffee. It was a liquid after all, it tasted good, and it gave me energy, or so I thought. I drank it in the morning and throughout my workday. Unfortunately, my thinking was dead wrong. Coffee is not the same as water because it dehydrates rather than hydrates your cells, and hydration is the key to life and to health.

On occasion, I'd substitute cola in place of the coffee. It was liquid after all, tasted good, and seemed effective at washing down burgers and fries. Plus, in a fast food place, there were free refills. If I was in a real hurry, I'd fill up my cup at the self-serve fountain, slurp it all down, and then refill it before going out the door. Most places offer a diet cola alternative. I avoided this because that stuff is made with artificial sweeteners, and I was pretty sure that those could be bad for me.

Cola without caffeine seemed unnatural as well. The caffeine was probably extracted with a number of unhealthy chemicals that could also be bad for me. I figured it was better to stick with the chemicals I knew, those I had read before on the side of cola cans, like ascorbic acid. I was fairly sure that the acid and all the other assorted chemicals were there for a good reason: to aid digestion.

I still had my coffee habit. One day though, I saw a patient who was drinking pots of coffee each day. He had multiple psychiatric symptoms including irritability, moodiness, anger issues, restlessness, and sleep problems. He had a hard time functioning due to anxiety and would have periodic panic attacks at work. He took anxiety medications to counteract the stimulant effect of the coffee. A light bulb went off in my head, and I realized I was performing the same pattern.

Determined to change, I resigned myself to cutting back on the caffeine. I'd go half-caf with my coffee. This seemed to be a good strategy, a baby step. I actually felt better having cut my caffeine intake. I was calmer, less irritable, and more effective in my work. Over time, I was able to transition to just 16 ounces of half-caf in the morning and de-caf only the rest of the day. I was down to the equivalent of one cup of caffeinated coffee a day and didn't feel the least bit deprived. I retained my habit of using half and half in my coffee, and over time this would become my only source of fat in the day. You do need some fat in your diet, after all.

Lastly, I became resigned to actually increasing my water intake. Water is necessary for life. Food is less important. I started drinking Crystal-Lite. It's a powdered, calorie free drink that mixes with water. I like the orange flavor. My wife bought a two-quart container with a tap that we kept in the refrigerator. I drank one full glass in the morning upon awakening and another while taking my morning vitamins. During my workday, I'd carry a water bottle and the portable Crystal-Lite tubes with me. I drank this throughout the day. My progress was obvious by the number of bathroom breaks I took, but in this case, more is better. Your body stays hydrated, and you're constantly flushing impurities from your system.

To this day, it's hard for me to drink straight, unflavored water. It simply has no taste. Drinking straight water is better if you can do it, but I've never turned the corner. I continue to get my 64-plus ounces daily in the form of decaf coffee and Crystal-Lite drink mix. I've eliminated soft drinks and virtually eliminated the caffeine. I feel much better, and you can too. Soft drinks and caffeinated coffee aren't listed in any of the food groups needed for good health. Neither counts towards your 64 ounces of water. It's for this reason that most people go through life dehydrated and this affects all aspects of your health. Decide right now to make a change. Choose a baby step and start doing it. Start making the changes and you'll begin to see the contrast between the old and new you.

List below the liquids you typically drink over the course of a day. ____

____

____

____

Now, estimate the daily amount of water you drink over the course of a day: _______oz. Can you do better than this?

A Note about Alcohol

I can't conclude the section on liquids without at least some mention of alcohol. In college I drank a lot, to the extent that it affected both my attendance and my grades.

Let me say it straight, underage drinking is just flat out dangerous. I learned the hard way. The part of the brain that controls judgment is not fully developed until after the teen years, so early alcohol use can negatively affect the process. Believe me, judgment is a necessary life-skill.

Today I drink red wine, one to two glasses a night and paired with dinner. Medical professionals seem to generally agree that light alcohol use daily has some heart healthy effects. This is the equivalent of one drink a day for women and two drinks a day for men. A drink means an ounce and a half of liquor, eight ounces of wine, or twelve ounces of beer.

Alcohol use in excess of the above amounts has been found to negatively affect a person's health. If you're of age and already drink, then observe the above guidelines. If you aren't already a drinker, don't start. Overall, the negative effects are likely to outweigh the positive ones, particularly when alcohol is used in excess. Alcohol use is especially risky if alcohol or drug addictions run in your family.

If there's some alcohol abuse in your family, taking the very first drink becomes a huge gamble. It's just not worth the risk since alcoholism runs in families, is progressive, debilitating, and chronic. Believe me, everyone who's been affected by it thought they could control their drinking. If you're an adult with the problem, immediately attend an Alcoholics Anonymous meeting, even if it's just to listen. Go to the Student Counseling Center if you're a college student with the problem, or talk it over with a trusted adult. I wish I would have received this help when I was eighteen or nineteen years old.

Something Old, Something New

There comes a time in your health journey, when you start to see the contrast between where you were and where you are now. It can be fairly dramatic. It becomes obvious in your belt size and the size of your clothes, and it can manifest itself in the change in your rituals.

My wife Pia and I had a Thursday night dining ritual for years. I would work one of my long unhealthy days, then drive a couple of hours home to meet my wife at our neighborhood bar and grill. We'd drink wine and talk about the week. It was sort of a debriefing session. Mostly, we'd eat unhealthy food that tasted really, really good.

The tavern burger and fries were standard. I had cheese, and she did without. We used lots of extra salt too, for the already salty food. Usually we had buffalo wings as well. To decrease the spiciness, I'd dip mine in the bleu cheese dressing. Of course, I needed more wine to wash down the wings. Occasionally, I'd have a side salad covered with more bleu cheese dressing. Heart surgeons know these choices are good for business.

Over time, I switched the bleu cheese to honey mustard, and later, to vinegar and oil. I weaned myself off those wings. Lastly, I cut out the tavern cheeseburger and fries. My wife and I decided to have a new meal on a regular basis. The wait staff took longer to adjust to it than we did. We really had turned the corner. We were on our way towards health.

We still met at our favorite place every Thursday. The time was the same, but we were very different. We'd start with a side salad without all the extras. Vinegar and oil as dressing made this even healthier. We changed our main course to blackened tuna steak with a baked potato (no sour cream). We still drank red wine during the meal, but less of it. This food was really good, plus it was healthy. We probably eliminated a hundred grams of fat and a couple thousand calories. Also, we had a lot less guilt after making the switch.

There will come a day when you, too, will look back at the old you in disbelief. To keep yourself on your path, make the changes gradually. Once you truly make the switch and establish healthy habits, going back won't be an option. You simply won't want to do it. Best of all, you'll have a hard time believing you ever lived that way in the first place. The new you will feel good, and the old you will be just wrong. Life is a marathon and with the new you, you'll finish strong. The old ways were killing you, and you'll discover this after the fact. You can transform your life and your health just like I did.

The Magic Jacket

When I was growing up, my dad owned a magic suit jacket. It fit every boy in our family, and it fit my dad too. This was very strange because we were all different sizes. As a teen, I was taller and leaner while my dad and brothers were shorter and stockier. Amazingly, the jacket would fit all of us for any formal type occasion. Clothes don't usually work this way. They're either tight or loose. Rarely do they fit just right.

When you've made up your mind to lose weight, there's usually that special jacket or pair of pants that you'd like to be able to wear again. It's an effort to get there. Every once in a while you try them on to measure your progress. If they're still tight, work some more. Try on those pants again in another month or two down the road. Eventually, as you lose weight and get healthier, there's hope that you'll be your old self at some point. The pants will fit when your body fits its frame.

My gauge of success was a belt. After five years I still wear it. It started at a size 41. This is the size for people who want to have heart attacks. I'd eat right and exercise and eventually I could go down a belt hole. Several months later, I'd drop another hole. Midway through the process, I had to get some new pants. This is both good and bad. The good part is the clear sign of progress. The bad part is the expense. If you're determined to reach your overall goal, buy cheap clothes, which are transition clothes only. You don't want to stay in them, and don't get too comfortable.

Several months and many healthy habits later, I dropped a couple more belt holes. This was more progress. Over an extended period of time, I dropped seven belt holes, or seven inches. I had to even add three holes to the belt because it didn't go thin enough.

A belt is a great measurement tool. I wear it all the time. It's a constant reminder of the size I used to be. Occasionally, I'll count the holes. This serves as a celebration and a deterrent, a reminder not to relapse into my old ways.

Lastly, put on the magic jacket or the magic pants, that special piece of clothing you couldn't let go of but never thought you'd wear again. Healthy habits truly do a body good. You, too, will get there, one inch at a time.

Don't feel like you have to do this all on your own. A family doctor or a drop-in clinic can be a great resource. They can encourage you, help you know your numbers, and offer preventative services to help you along the way. A personal trainer or health coach can also get you started or even motivate you once you get further along. Now describe your magic jacket. What item of clothing will be your gauge of success?

Inside Out

While some jackets are magic there are others that are reversible. You know, the kind that looks good both inside and outside? Have you ever owned one? I had one once and both sides always looked good. Health isn't the same way. On the surface you can look good. Your weight might be adequate and you have decent muscle tone. On the inside it could be a different story. You could be building up plaque in your arteries, your blood pressure could be up, and your blood sugars could be getting out of whack. You could be dying from the inside out.

People who swear off doctors never see the inside of that jacket. They're never aware of problems that are developing. They judge their health by the surface only, not knowing what's underneath. An iceberg looks harmless enough from the top, but it's the 80 percent underwater that sinks the ship. It's time for you to be proactive with your health. You need to know both the outside and the inside story. Only with knowledge can you take the steps to improve the outcome. Putting your head in the sand like an ostrich is not helpful, and extreme doctor avoidance could kill you.

The old phrase, "You can't judge a book by its cover," still holds true today. Commit to finding out what's going on beneath the surface. Some of the healthiest looking gym junkies could die tomorrow. Plaque could break off an artery and lead to an immediate heart attack just because they never bothered to look good on the inside.

Drive-By-Docs

Family doctors are really great and I'm convinced that everybody should have one. These are folks who come to know you over the years, understand your problems, and can coordinate specialty care if you ever need it. The problem today is that they just don't stay with it as long as they used to. My doctor, Steve Karem, M.D., in Floyds Knobs, Indiana, is very stable, but nowadays he might be the exception rather than the rule. I bet I've seen Steve for ten years and he's truly an awesome doctor. My wife Pia, however, has had four doctors in four years. Her doctors have been victims of burnout, corporate buyouts, disillusionment, and insurance disputes. Each time my wife is forced to switch doctors, she has to go through the whole initial work-up thing, various tests, and paperwork, only to have to do it again one year later. It's aggravating to say the least. Then, if she would get sick, her doctors were often too busy to work her into their schedule due to corporate productivity, lack of appointment availability, and other excuses.

Another option is using drive-by-docs. It's a great concept to offer medical services in people's neighborhoods right where they shop and where they get their medicines. I've been very impressed with a couple of clinics in my town. The first is inside a national grocery store chain and the other is in a national drugstore chain. Both are staffed by nurse practitioners, who seem very competent and very professional. You don't even need an appointment and typically there's not much of a wait. These are great resources to use if you come down with an infection, feel under the weather, or need something like an antibiotic prescribed. I've had great experiences at both places, and it's a fraction of the cost of an immediate care type clinic. I'm sure costs vary but my visits have cost from $50 to $75 plus they're willing to bill your insurance. Also, if you pay cash, I think there might be a discount.

The other thing I do to manage health care costs is to use medications from the discount list. I'll typically print the discount lists for large pharmacy chains from the Internet and take them with me to the appointment. I always ask the nurse practitioner to try something from the list unless it's simply not a medication that's going to help. These drugs are offered at great discounts, around $10 to $14 for a three-month supply. In my work, I tell the patients that I evaluate to do the same thing. Too often, doctors and nurse practitioners prescribe medications based upon drug rep marketing without thinking about the cost to the patient. There are times when people simply go without medications once they learn what they will cost. Don't be one of these people. If medicines are prescribed, there's usually a reason.

If you live in a metro area, do some research and see if some of these clinics are around you. Check them out in advance and become familiar with what they can offer. That way, when you are truly sick and need help, you can be seen without too much delay. A quick start of an antibiotic can often keep a small infection from getting a whole lot worse while you're trying to get seen in a traditional doctor's office.

Proactive Prevention

My guess is that you're a driver and that you probably change the oil in your car regularly. The quick oil change people say to do it every three thousand miles. Maybe you do it every five thousand. The point is that you do it, and you do it to prevent bigger and more costly problems with your car. These quick-change places also do a 20-30 point safety check while they have your car in there. They might find your air filter clogged, loose belts, or even dangerously worn tires. Again, addressing these problems now will save you time and money in the long run. Likewise, your body is a vehicle and has to carry you through life. Shouldn't you treat it with at least the same care you give your car?

Preventative maintenance is always a good idea starting with an annual physical exam. This is relatively painless and doesn't even take that long. The doctor will check your heart, your lungs, blood pressure, reflexes, and for men, the prostate. This PSA test helps rule out developing prostate problems. Typically, a staff person will draw some blood and have you urinate in a cup. My doctor has a door you put the cup in and it magically disappears into the urine analysis room. Usually a blood panel is run with results sent to you later. There's also typically a cardiac risk profile done that looks at your good and bad cholesterol along with your triglycerides. These results show blood sugar levels and red and white blood cell counts as well. If a problem is identified, it can be dealt with while it's still minor.

Men are really bad about going to doctors. I'm not sure if they're scared of what they might find or if they're just plain stubborn. Women are usually more sensible about prevention. They don't mind a periodic check-up and are even willing to see a doctor when they're sick. Many men prefer to suffer and tough it out, as if they're invincible. It's no wonder that women live longer than men and men with women in their lives live longer than those without women. Funny how that works, isn't it?

The next thing is to take advantage of companies that offer multiple health screenings all at one time, something I try to do every year or two. Some set up a clinic in a local church and others might use a mobile medical van in the parking lot of a big-box store. These companies do thousands of dollars worth of screening tests for around $270. This is a fantastic service and another one of those that could potentially identify life changing health problems while they're still small and treatable. My tests included a cholesterol profile including triglycerides, BP, heart rate, bone density, peripheral artery disease testing, carotid artery screening, and screening for aortic aneurysm. Also included was a screening for arterial stiffness, an echocardiogram, and an EKG of the heart. A number of these are Doppler studies that would cost thousands of dollars in a normal medical diagnostic facility. Results come to you a few weeks later in the mail and a copy is sent to your doctor by your request.

I highly advise that you watch for this service advertised in your community or simply go online to find out when these companies will be in your area. Believe me, this is money well spent. After all, an ounce of prevention is worth a pound of cure. Spend the money. You and your vehicle are worth it. Once you get broken down, things become a whole lot more expensive.

3. CHANGING FROM THE OUTSIDE IN
The Food Diary

ONCE YOU COMMIT to traveling the road to health, you'll want to keep a food diary. Like the exercise journal, this gives you a baseline of where you're starting. Date the page and make entries each day. If your diet is horrible, that's OK—just record it. Write down every food you eat for breakfast, lunch, and dinner, as well as any foods you eat in between. You should record evening snacks as well. Be honest and accurate for at least a week. This is your starting point. Don't change anything right off. Just figure out where you are right now with this snapshot of your current habits.

Include everything you eat or drink throughout the day from the time you get up until the time you go to bed. Record the whole week as I suggested. Using the concept of a stoplight, list your foods under red, yellow, or green. Red is for stop. This is a food you shouldn't eat much. Yellow means caution. This food is OK if eaten occasionally and in the proper serving size. Green is for go. This is a food that's good for you, is part of a healthy diet, and should be eaten regularly and in the suggested number of servings, such as fruits and vegetables, 5-9 servings a day, grains 9-11 daily. Just use your own judgment when assigning the color category because at this point, you're just trying to create awareness.

The Harvard Food Pyramid is an excellent guide to the number of servings you should get from each food group each day. I suggest you Google this on-line, print the image you like, and post it on your refrigerator. Try to use it daily and get used to counting your servings from each food group each day. See if you've gone over the recommended servings. Again, all of this is just to create awareness. You haven't made any changes just yet.

Think about how you were feeling as you ate. Write down your feelings. Highlight any feelings other than hunger, since you should only eat when you're hungry. Unfortunately, many of us eat out of boredom, anxiety, or frustration. This is something you'll want to change. Most couch eating isn't related to hunger. Try to eat most of your food at a table, like the early pioneers did.

Lastly, you should record whatever you drink each day. Water is the best fluid. Eight glasses a day or 64 ounces is the minimum. Highlight everything you drink besides water. Too much soda can erode your tooth enamel. If you have to drink it, make sure it's sugar free and caffeine free. Excess coffee can cause anxiety and contribute to nervous eating. Fruit juice is all right, but only in small amounts. For example, juice like orange juice, is high sugar and calories. It's better to eat an orange or an apple than to drink the juice, so that way you're not cheating yourself out of the fiber.

Decide to shake things up a little after you've done your first one-week analysis. Make a small change at first, something that will give you success. Maybe you drink more water or cut out some soda. Maybe you cut out pork bacon and switch to low fat turkey bacon. You might even decrease your caffeine intake, add more veggies, or eat more fruit. Dairy is important too. Are you getting enough of it (3 servings a day)? Continue your food diary for several weeks, and make healthy modifications to your diet each time you review the previous week. Eventually, you'll want to be eating according to the Harvard

Food Pyramid, drinking enough water, and eating only when hungry and not out of boredom or frustration.

After a couple months of transforming your diet, the food log will be unnecessary, since you will have established new and healthier habits. Your body will be able to tell what's good by the reaction to the food and how well you feel. You'll feel a lot better about yourself and the new road you've taken. At that point, you can practice the 80/20 rule. Make the right food choice four out of five times. Don't punish yourself if you don't. If you're exercising and eating right there are times you can treat yourself and not feel bad about it. Several times a year, I eat a tavern burger with cheese just because I get the urge. Sometimes I'll even eat fried chicken. That's OK. I count that in the 20 percent. Most of the time I eat grilled or baked fish, chicken, or turkey.

If you're at a birthday party, it's all right to eat the cake. Being healthy shouldn't include feeling deprived or punished. Feel good about what you're doing and allow for some variation.

Eating Out

In today's fast paced world, people eat out a lot and that's fine. You just have to learn to make good choices. I've come a long way in my choices since choosing health. In the past, breakfast would be biscuits and gravy and dinner out would be country-fried steak. My mom loved this stuff, and I didn't have the heart to let her eat it alone.

Today, eating out can mean eating healthy. Choosing baked/grilled foods rather than fried foods is a major step and immediately puts you on the right track. Turkey, chicken, and fish can all be ordered this way. You'll be surprised how good these foods can taste, and you'll be substantially decreasing your fat grams.

Secondly, make a decision to eliminate things that are creamy, like Alfredo sauce, dressings like ranch and bleu cheese, sour cream, tartar sauce, and mayonnaise. These are all high fat, high calorie, and detract from your overall health. Salads sound healthy, but deluxe salads with dressings are loaded with both fat and calories. Eggs, croutons, bacon bits, and cheese crumbles all detract from what once was healthy: the greens. Choose spinach salad or salad greens rather than iceberg lettuce, since iceberg lettuce is mostly water. The darker the lettuce the better it is for you. Top it off with vinegar and oil, fat-free Italian, or fat-free honey mustard as the least of the evils.

Portion control is also important when eating out. Remember to put half your order in a to-go box before you start to eat. Most restaurant portions are three times what you should eat. Resist the temptation of dessert if possible. Adding dessert can destroy all the other good choices you made in the course of the meal. If you must have it, try having fruit, Jell-O, fat-free pudding, sherbet, or a small scoop of low-fat ice cream. Double chocolate brownie supreme, or Italian cream cake will make you feel really guilty afterwards.

Maintaining better awareness will help you when eating out in both restaurants and in drive-thru's. Drive-thru food requires making common sense choices as well. Grilled vs. fried is always good. Hold back ordering all of the extra sauces that destroy an otherwise healthy meal. Skip the fries altogether and watch the fat grams. Taco Bell has Fresco style food that eliminates creamy ingredients, making the items have only 5-9 grams of fat. Subway has sandwiches with 6 grams of fat or less as long as you don't ruin them by adding mayo and fatty dressings. Even McDonald's has healthy options on the menu. Find a healthy choice you like and stick with it. I'm hooked on the Taco Bell ninety-nine cent chicken burrito, Fresco style. It's both healthy and filling and causes me no guilt whatsoever. At McDonald's I opt for the grilled chicken honey mustard snack wrap and a side salad.

Again, try to observe the 80/20 rule. Make the right choice four out of five times, knowing that the other 20 percent of the time, it's OK to treat yourself. A small bag of fries on occasion or an ice cream sundae won't be the end of the world. Enjoy!

Portion Distortion

Today I'm on a mission trip at a Guatemalan orphanage. Hogar Rafael Ayau in Guatemala City is home to 30-40 children. The kids are happy and healthy and have weight proportionate to their height. What a great concept. This is my third trip and I'm always impressed with the way the kids eat. They eat a variety of foods, but just one portion each. One serving of each food is all that you need. It's really enough for what your body requires. In America, excess has become the norm and super-sized meals have become expected.

If you're an American, you're likely eating portions three times what is needed to fuel your body. Unfortunately, this happens both at home and in restaurants. Just for kicks, read the serving size on food containers. A half cup is usually standard. Try measuring the food you are served on a typical dinner plate. You'll be shocked. It's so much more than what you need.

In the Guatemalan orphanage where I am, most of the kids look lean and healthy. They've never had the super-size-me mentality. They eat the single portion sizes that are served to them and are more than content. You can do it, too. It's a matter of awareness, first, and changing your habits second.

Once you gain awareness about the number of servings you're eating, then you can make some adjustments. A serving size for most foods is a half-cup. Gradually reduce your portions so that you're eating just one portion of each food served. Over time, your stomach will adjust to the change and you'll feel satisfied with this amount.

America is a great country, but we definitely live in a land of excess. In Guatemala, people eat what they can afford, which is generally a serving size of each food. Eating more food just because it's available is not better. In this case, less is really more.

Muscle Mass

In middle age, weird things start to happen. Hair grows where it shouldn't, you have to go to the bathroom several times a night, and you can pull a muscle just by taking a shower. Something else happens around this time. You start to lose muscle mass. Muscles in your body start to break down and deteriorate. This is bad because muscles are needed for strength and movement. They also burn lots more calories than other body tissue. Less muscle means a decreased metabolism and more calories going to fat rather than being burned.

I'm not advocating that you become a muscle-head or a gym rat. You simply need to do some weight bearing exercise in your middle years and beyond. This could be a 20-30 minute weight routine two or three days a week. A gym workout is fine, but you can also use dumbbells right in your home. Get a mixed set of pairs from 2.5 to 25 pounds. Start out light with a weight you can manage 12 times each. To maintain muscle and tone, lighter weights are OK. To build muscle you want to use a weight you can lift eight times before exhaustion.

The following exercises are recommended, provided you have no medical restrictions. You can purchase exercise journals to record your workouts or simply print workout logs off the Internet.

- Chest press
- Shoulder press
- Lat pull-downs
- Chest Fly
- Triceps curl
- Biceps curl

- Ball squats
- Calf raises
- Abdominal crunches
- Leg extensions, Leg press, Leg curls

Google these on the Internet and then print out the instructions. This will help you start out doing each exercise with the right form. You can probably look these up on YouTube and watch a video clip of how they're actually performed.

The reps should be slow and deliberate. Focus your attention on the muscles you're trying to work. Don't rush! Gym rats make this mistake all the time. Faster and jerkier is not better. Lift to a count of two and release to a count of two. All of these exercises can be done right in your home with dumbbells, a chair, a bench, or the floor. As you age, maintaining muscle is very important. It preserves strength, mobility and helps your balance. Your metabolism will run at a higher rate and physically you'll just feel better.

A proper routine will work arm and leg muscles along with the large muscle groups in your back and your chest. Additionally, you'll need to focus on working the core muscles in your trunk. These are strengthened by a variety of exercises including crunches, sit-ups, side crunches, bicycle kicks, and by using a balance board.

Core muscles are really important for balance. Falls are the most common cause of injuries as people age and improved balance helps prevent falls. Good balance is critical to other life areas as well beyond just the physical aspects.

Supplements

My mom, Joy Oetken, was one of the finest people you'd ever meet. She went to church often. She was always helping others. Mom didn't want any recognition for it. She was simply playing the role of a servant like Jesus did. Mom was doing WWJD before the trendy bracelets ever came out. She was a real angel on earth.

Mom had a poor diet. To keep going, she drank lots of coffee and took supplements. You had to be cautious when opening her kitchen cabinets, since she stashed all of her supplements in the cabinet with the coffee cups. It was risky to open that cabinet. Either coffee cups or supplements would come tumbling down. I came to believe that Paisley Road in Louisville was the epicenter of supplement science.

The National Enquirer was one of Mom's news sources about supplements. She also relied on infomercials and word of mouth. Each morning, Mom would take a swig of vinegar right out of the bottle, which she was convinced was good for everything. Next, she'd take some garlic tablets and later some fish oil. By noon, the smell of salad oozed from her pores and was detectable from thirty feet away. At one point, she may have been taking as many as twenty supplements; saw palmetto, niacin, red rice yeast, St. John's Wort, oyster shell, among others. Smoking three packs of cigarettes a day, Mom had to take "real" medicine as well. This was prescribed for the Chronic Obstructive Pulmonary Disease (COPD), which would eventually kill her.

If your house has a weak foundation, you can't shore it up by painting the gutters. Supplements can never take the place of a healthy, active lifestyle and a healthy diet. The primary goal of companies that make dietary supplements is to make money. You won't find this in their mission statements. Essentially, it's an unregulated industry. While some of the stuff might actually be good for you, each bottle has a disclaimer marked in small print at the bottom of the label. It reads something like this, "This product makes no claim to diagnose, cure or decrease any specific medical illness or medical symptoms. Claims regarding the effectiveness of this product are not endorsed by the FDA. This product is not a substitute for a well balanced diet."

Having been raised by an alternative medicine guru, I couldn't help but adopt some of Mom's techniques. Slowly, I added one supplement or another for various medical conditions. Before I knew it, I was taking around twelve supplements. I took each one for specific problems I self-diagnosed, and I took some for prevention purposes. In the meanwhile, I continued my unhealthy lifestyle, so I was probably doing more harm than good. It's hard to know exactly what the supplements do to your system and even harder to know what the interaction effects are. Unlike traditional medicines, these interaction effects are largely unstudied. I was probably supplementing myself to death and still doing all the wrong things.

As I added healthy habits to my lifestyle, I decided to decrease my supplements. A well-balanced, high fiber, low fat diet takes care of most of your nutritional needs. Whatever you're lacking at that point can be taken care of with a multi-vitamin. Simpler is usually better. My new regimen consists of fish oil twice a day for heart health, Glucosamine twice a day for joint health (after age forty), a multi-vitamin in the morning, an 81 mg aspirin and an over-the-counter allergy pill once a day (Loritadine 10 mg) so I can live with cats. I'm convinced that this is much better for me, and it's a regimen that I can manage. There was a period when I took at least five supplements for cholesterol alone. When you get to this point just give in and take the statin medication from your doctor. These medicines are getting cheaper all the time, including Lipitor. They work and they work fast.

At age 52, I feel better than I have felt in my entire life. I'm not supplement free, but I'm close to it. I'm not drinking vinegar from the bottle, nor am I taking garlic, saw palmetto, or oyster shells. My vitamins primarily come from the foods I eat. Whatever nutrients I lack are made up by the multi-vitamin I take. I'm saving a lot of money by just eating the right food and I'm saving a lot of time by not worrying about when and how much of each of the multiple supplements to take. The bonus is that I've eliminated the potential harm that could come from mixing all those supplements without any clear guidelines.

My mom died in her sixties largely because of her unhealthy lifestyle. Believe me, massive amounts of supplements are not the answer. Keep it simple. Eat the right stuff with lots of variety and you'll get most of the vitamins you need the natural way.

Is It Greek To You?

Lots of research suggests that the key to health and longevity is the reverse of the American way. Americans eat high fat, low fiber diets when they should do the opposite. A low fat, high fiber diet is actually what's required. It's what your body was designed to process. Additionally, it's the diet found in Mediterranean countries where people live long lives. Heart disease was not imported. It was patented in America before it was exported around the world by fast food corporations.

Fad diets are short lived and fade away. You've heard all of them: the Atkins diet, the Abs diet, the South Beach diet, the Pritikin diet, Oprah's diet. They fade in and out of popularity like fashion trends. People that practice these are on a constant yo-yo of weight loss and weight gain. It might even be better just to be overweight than constantly going back and forth, which can't be good for the system. Eating like a Mediterranean is a doable life-style. It simply involves gradually changing your food choices to those things that are healthier.

What is it? Good question. It's a lifestyle based upon eating more fish and less red meat. Fish oil can also be used. Both give you omega three fatty acids that are good for both heart health and digestion. Eating more fiber is important, too. This requires choosing whole grains and brown rice rather than processed grains. One hundred percent whole wheat bread takes the place of white bread and brown rice replaces white rice. Other fiber sources include lots of fruits and vegetables, at least five to nine servings a day. These can be very filling and help cure both the vitamin deficiencies and the fiber efficiencies that people typically have. There's virtually no limit on vegetable intake.

Variety is the key! Not all fruits and vegetables are created equal. Different colored produce have different nutrients. If you choose different colors it's like taking a multiple vitamin with fiber added. Take potatoes for example. A sweet potato is far more nutritious than a white potato and has more fiber. Dark green veggies like spinach and kale are thought to have anti-cancer properties. Tomatoes contain lycopine, which is also thought to prevent a number of diseases. In the area of fruits, an apple a day keeps the doctor away, but a pear keeps him away for longer. The fiber content of pears is much higher and is beneficial in helping to clean out your system. Try to eat whole fruits and vegetables if possible and eat them more often. Juice is not bad, but it's typically high calorie and low fiber. Find some things you like and resolve to eat them.

Mediterranean people also eat beneficial oils. Olive oil has a number of health promoting properties. At most meals, you can season olive oil with spices and dip whole grain bread into it. Use this oil for cooking and in salad dressings whenever possible. Eating fish several times a week can give you the beneficial fish oil you need, but most Americans probably need a supplement. Fish oil supplements using wild salmon are typically the best and have the least mercury contamination. Two thousand mcu's is recommended, which is usually 2-3 capsules daily. Put the container in your freezer and take the frozen capsules in the morning and at night. This eliminates the fishy taste some people otherwise belch up. If you take one mid-day away from home, opt for the coated caplets.

Wine also tends to be part of life in the Mediterranean part of the world. Many studies suggest that alcohol use, one to two drinks a day, has some heart benefits. Specifically, red wine is high in antioxidants and flavenols. These substances fight free radicals in the body that destroy cells. Red wine in moderation also raises the good HDL cholesterol level in your body. The HDL cleans your vascular system acting like a Roto-Rooter for your arteries. It counteracts the LDL bad cholesterol that is attracted to your artery walls. Wine is also an anti-anxiety agent, which may have some benefit in itself. In Mediterranean countries, wine is used at meals with friends and family, further adding the healthful properties of having social networks.

The people in this part of the world eat more often than Americans, but generally eat the right things. Eating smaller meals more often is preferable to eating three large meals a day. They tend to drink more water, too, which helps all systems of the body. Unlike hard driving, type-A Americans, people of the Mediterranean show joy in their work, in their families, and at meals. They express emotions that Americans usually repress. When they get tired, they nap; they're like cats in this regard. Mid-afternoon is naptime. Shops close. Business people go home. They lunch and nap. Maybe they start working again around 6PM and eat much later at 9 or 10 o'clock. Rest is important for people everywhere, particularly people who are under a lot of stress.

Ironically, the Mediterranean diet isn't a diet at all. It's a change in habits and in lifestyle. Obviously, you can't change your entire culture, but you can personally change the foods you eat, when you eat them, how often, how much, whom you eat with, and what you drink. You can also resign yourself to walking longer distances, like people in other parts of the world. You can become more expressive and not bottle up negative emotions and can choose to rest when you're tired, even if it's for brief catnaps. Eat more fish, as well as more fruits and veggies. Add olive oil and maybe even red wine to your diet and eat whole grains. Choose foods from all the food groups including dairy. Most importantly, try to limit your fat intake.

The Mediterranean way is the way of health and longevity. After all, these are the folks who started running marathons before running was even cool. Try to be more Mediterranean. Your body will thank you. You'll have better health and you'll demonstrate good habits for your family. The end results will be so much better as you do more of the right things and put more of the right stuff in your body. Before moving on, complete the following statement: I resolve to incorporate some aspects of the Mediterranean lifestyle into my life by: _________

____

____

____

____

Cats and Toilet Paper

I was around the age of 40 when I lost two dogs in a divorce. I avoided grocery stores because the amount of choices overwhelmed me. My primary food shopping was at K-Mart where there were only two aisles of food. This was simpler, and it didn't short-circuit my ADHD brain. I had to learn to survive physically and emotionally. My therapist prescribed a cat.

"What no drugs? No Prozac?" I asked. She said a cat would help me heal.

A patient of mine gave me a stray cat from her farm in Georgetown, Indiana. I named the cat Georgia. Sometimes I used the more formal name, Miss Georgia. She was good medicine for me. On a bad night, I'd lie on the couch and cry. Miss Georgia lay on my chest, licked my face, and purred. It was very comforting. She sensed my moods and gave me just the right amount of attention. I'm pretty sure she could live without me, but the reverse wasn't true. Miss Georgia was good therapy.

Cats are far from needy. They're clean, independent, and unlike people they seem to know what's good for them. They like sunshine, naps, occasional exercise, and stretching. When they need affection, they ask for it. What a concept.

Most impressive, however, is how clean cats are. Miss Georgia was snow white with a little black on her face and some black on her paws. When not resting or bolting frantically around the house, she was busy cleaning her fur. Cats are cleaner than some people. Without fail, she did her business in the litter box down in the basement. The process was quick, clean, and efficient, unlike some people who go in the bathroom and don't come out for an hour. Georgia's tail end was clean without any help from me. It was all about the food.

Cats eat the right stuff. It's specifically formulated for their bodies and attempts to simulate their natural diet. Other animals are the same. Have you ever seen rabbit droppings or deer droppings? Most animals eat what their bodies were made to eat, unless they're corrupted by humans. Rabbits don't need toilet paper and neither do deer. Your hunter/gatherer ancestors probably didn't need it either. They ate lots of fiber, which made elimination quick, clean, and efficient for them too. Today humans use lots of toilet paper and even clog toilets with it.

Certainly, elimination isn't a pretty topic, but it's a measure of the quality of your diet. There's a saying attached to computers that says, "garbage in – garbage out." This applies to humans as well. If you struggle to do your business, then your body's trying to tell you something. If your TP use is resulting in the destruction of forests, then it's time to change. A trip to Europe is instructive in this regard. There, the used TP goes in the can next to the commode. Europeans eat healthier than Americans and usually can get by with two pieces. Resign yourself to do better! Fiber, fiber, and more fiber is good for your pipes.

Unfortunately, the smelly truth is that the quality of your diet is reflected in the quality of your poop. There's no pretty way to say it. Like most Americans, you're probably fiber deficient. Fiber is the plumber for your pipes. It's your personal Roto-Rooter. It cleans your arteries, and it cleans your colon. Have you ever heard of a cat coming down with colon cancer, prostate cancer, stomach cancer or rectal cancer?

Let's face the facts. You are what you eat. Why shouldn't you be at least as healthy as a house pet? A number of us will suffer life-changing medical problems that are largely self-inflicted. You can do better. Strive for better poop. More fiber, more movement, and more water are the three key ingredients. Before reading on, complete the following statement: I will add more fiber to my diet by: __________

____

____

____

____

Walking and Talking

Running a psychology consulting business with numerous employees requires lots of phone calls at times. In my early health transformation, I decided to make these while walking. I'd drive to the local park, put on my walking shoes, and cover a mile loop two times. During the first loop, I returned phone calls and initiated calls as well, trying to take care of business. The second loop I walked at a UPS driver's pace. I could take a call if I got one, but the talking would be a bigger effort.

Walking is not only great for the body; it's also great for the mind. It can be almost meditative in a way, helping to clear out the mental cobwebs. You can do self-talk during the process and repeat your personal affirmation as you walk. You can get into a rhythmic cadence with your steps and talk to God if you want. Mentally, you can reflect on the things you're doing right and the things you need to change. Spiritual masters have walked the labyrinth for years for these same reasons.

Walking can be fun too! There's no special equipment required. You can walk right out your door and just take off for 30-40 minutes. Develop a standard route, and then vary it when you get bored. Add variety like a local zoo walk, a park path, or a walk through your favorite part of town. I live in the Highlands of Louisville, which is very walkable. I hop a bus towards downtown and then walk back along Bardstown Road. I look in store windows, people watch, and sample coffee shops along the way. It's a great way to exercise, and I try to make it fun.

Winter walking is also OK, provided you bundle up for it. You might also walk the local malls, or even the perimeters of a Wal-Mart, Lowes, or Home Depot store. This allows you to get your shopping in during the same trip. Try to buy something to justify using their space. Some cities even have downtown skyway connectors that allow you to walk long distances without ever going outside. Downtown medical complexes are like this as well.

Remember your daily step goal is 10,000. Extra walking will be required. Make sure to wear your pedometer. If you're just starting out, keep an exercise log for encouragement. Remember, your body was made to walk about five to ten miles a day. You can do this and it will be one of the best habits you ever develop. My amazing neighbor did it until she was 92-years-old. How's that for a testimonial?

My Amazing Neighbor

When you've lived in a lot of houses like I have, you get to experience all kinds of neighbors. At my first house, I had a skill-saw-possessed neighbor named Roger. He was a good neighbor, but he ran that skill saw 24/7. His wife Cindy was a saint. On the other side were Dick and Gail. They were great, down-to-earth people. They liked me until I was confused about the property line. I accidentally cut down their maple tree and a fence went up shortly thereafter. I couldn't blame them. I've run into Gail occasionally at the coffee shop. She's either forgiven me or hides it well.

In the metropolis of Hopkinsville, Kentucky, I ended up with a redneck wife-beater on one side and a truck driver/mechanic on the other side. Some mechanics like to work in their backyards at night with spotlights and feel the need to rev their engines to remind you that they're mechanics. This could go on late into the night. Beer seemed to help them focus on their work. In a neighborhood, backyard mechanics don't work alone. They need an audience. The helpers drink beer, cuss about women, spit, and occasionally hand tools to the mechanic. I guess it's a good life as long as you're not the neighbor.

My recent and hopefully my last neighbor is the amazing one. She lives alone. Up until just last year, she drove "old" people to doctor's appointments. Corinne had worked at the local psychiatric hospital gift shop and she had donated some time at our local art museum. She also did some volunteer work with the Helping Hand Ministries, which serves Appalachia. She still plays cards with friends, and kept up with her e-mail until recently. Not long ago, she got a different car because the old one was acting up. If she had extra time, she would visit an old person in a nursing home. At the age of 93, she finally stopped driving.

Corinne was an amazing neighbor. I hope you have one like her yourself. She's 95-years-young as this book goes to print. Recently, she took Tylenol for foot pain but had never used an over the counter pain pill before in her life. Within the last year, Corinne took an antibiotic, also a new experience for her. Until just recently, she lived alone, cared for her house, managed her finances, and did her own grocery shopping. She'd take out her own garbage, but Hugh, the eighty-seven year old neighbor across the street likes the exercise, so he does that task for her. Corinne had always stayed active and even now she maintains a positive attitude in spite of recent chronic pain from sciatica.

As a child, her family had a summer home in J-town, Kentucky. Today it's a suburb, but at the time it was pure country. Recently, she told me she and her siblings would ride their bikes out there to get around for the summer. Corinne road her bike ten miles on what was a rough gravel road with grass growing in the middle. She and her siblings rode their bikes all around the area, they swam in the Chenoweth Run Creek, and they played outdoors constantly. At the end of the summer, they would ride their bikes down that long gravel road back to their Highlands neighborhood. Today, this would be a difficult bike ride. On a gravel road, the difficulty factor would increase tenfold. Corinne was active as a child, and she stayed very active up until the last year or two.

In Louisville, we've had some really strange weather. One week I believe in global warming, but the next week I believe in global cooling. Over the past year, we've had two severe windstorms and one severe ice storm. Lots of trees and tree limbs came down as the result. The other folks in our neighborhood were none too eager to start the clean-up process. Insurance claims would need to be filed, adjustors would have to come out, and then they'd have to hire workers. Corinne wasn't like the other neighbors. She got out there the next day and started picking up sticks and other debris.

Corinne patrolled her yard, searching for sticks big and small. She'd stoop over, pick up a stick then repeat the pattern until she had an armful. She'd stack them in neat piles, and then eventually carry them to the street. Some, she'd stuff in her yard waste can and haul it out. She hired some men to do the big limbs only, the ones that required chainsaws. Stooping and getting back up was good for her, and she enjoyed being outside. If she tired, she'd simply rest and then start again. Corinne could have afforded to have someone do all the work, but that would have cheated her out of exercise. She simply wouldn't have that.

Up until just a couple years ago, my amazing neighbor walked about two miles a day. She'd put on her sunglasses, grab her cane, and head down the street. She walked at a good pace with a hunched over posture. I think her back was OK at the time. She was simply determined to focus her attention on the ground. The last thing she wanted was to fall and break her hip. That would make her like the other old people in the nursing homes. She walked daily from her house in the neighborhood up to the main road, Bardstown Road. It's about a mile each way. I made sure there was a bench at the half way mark. Occasionally, Corinne might rest a bit before proceeding onward. She'd chat with people along the way. What a remarkable lady.

Corinne knew the benefit of staying active. After all, she was still taking her walks at age 93 and had no health issues yet. When the weather was bad, she rode her exercise bike on the sun-porch. She'd stay busy moving about the house, dusting, cleaning, washing the china, polishing silver and other chores. Her friends from the old folk's homes would call and she'd chat with them. Sometimes, they'd call, needing rides somewhere and she'd oblige them.

Being active throughout life had preserved Corinne's health. Maybe she had good genes as well. She enjoyed a good quality of life because of her healthy habits. What a testament to being active. Would you rather spend your later years being independent or lying in some facility with people telling you when to eat, drink, and use the bathroom? Corinne chose health, and you can too!

Only recently, she's needed help at the age of 95. Living to a ripe old age is only desirable if you've maintained your health. It's no fun being sick, frail, and fragile. Make the right choices now, so you can have the benefits not just now but later. My amazing neighbor made the right choices and has been able to enjoy her senior years as the result. You can do it too if you develop healthy habits now as an investment in your future.

Update: Corinne has now passed away. She was 95 years and 8-months old when she died. Corinne was able to die with dignity in her home with family and friends by her side. She spent virtually no time in a hospital nor did she ever need nursing home care. She was a blessing to be around and truly was an amazing neighbor. I'm confident she'll be an amazing angel as well.

Life—Up In Smoke

No book on health should leave out a basic lecture on the perils of tobacco use. This one is no different. If you smoke or one of your loved ones smokes, read on. If you don't, feel free to skip to the next section.

I grew up in a house with a mom who smoked like a chimney. Pall Malls were her brand. They were rated way up there for tar and nicotine levels. Mom was frugal, so she wanted to get her money's worth. Even the secondhand smoke was powerful. The house was thick with it. The nicotine stained the curtains, the ceilings, the walls, and the wallpaper. Chronic exposure to the smoke caused her dog Ruffy to develop a smoker's cough.

Mom loved those cigarettes as much as she loved her children: Dave, Todd, Dan, Lynnie, Kevin, Kerri and me, Chris. In fact, she said she couldn't have raised seven kids without them. From time to time she'd send the tobacco companies thank you notes for spending money to refute the government's false claims that cigarettes were bad for you. She developed a three pack a day, chain-smoking habit. Mom was absolutely convinced that the government manipulated all the studies saying smoking caused cancer.

Over the years, Mom started to have coughing fits where she just couldn't get her breath. She'd cough "gunk" out of her lungs. She struggled to breathe at times. The doctors had warned her, but she lived in denial. At some point in her early 60s she was diagnosed with COPD/Emphysema. It's a chronic and progressive lung problem that gets worse and leads to death.

In Mom's case, it got worse just as predicted, yet she continued to smoke. It got harder and harder for her to breathe. She ended up on ten or more different medicines and breathing treatments each day. Mom was in the hospital on oxygen at times. She'd pull the tubes from her nose and go smoke in the bathroom. Talk about a serious addiction!

Eventually, the next diagnosis came. She had lung cancer, the biggie, and she had part of her lung surgically removed. Mom was a fighter; she'd bounce back, and then go downhill again. Throughout her medical ordeal, she kept smoking. During her last several months, I had the privilege of managing her daily medications. Since the regimen got to be so huge, she just couldn't keep up with it on her own. I enjoyed the contact with her and the conversation. She had lots of life wisdom to share. Her faith kept her going and she had no fear. She knew exactly where she was headed. She taught me to live in the moment.

Mom eventually died of Emphysema at age 68, ten years before the predicted life expectancy for a female. She cheated herself out of those years, and she cheated those who loved her out of them as well. Her lungs slowly filled with fluid, she needed in-home oxygen, and she couldn't even walk across the room without getting winded. It was a bad way to go, since she suffocated and drown at the same time.

Mom died at home. She was on her favorite couch with her dog Ruffy by her side. I know my mom went directly to heaven, since she was an angel even on earth. She helped so many people and could have helped even more if her life wasn't cut short. Before Mom died, she scribbled, "Work on Earth is done" on a piece of paper.

Mom's dog Ruffy moved to my brother Dave's home, which is a nonsmoking environment, and the dog's smoker's cough cleared up.

My brother put her on a health regimen and even started feeding her dog food. She's still alive today.

You can change too. The lungs start to repair themselves within only months after you stop smoking. There are so many resources available today to help you quit. If you're not inclined to quit for yourself, then quit for your family. What my siblings and I went through with our mother was horrible, plus, we were robbed of ten years of time with her. Do you want to wish this on your loved ones? Just think about it.

Make up your mind to quit and set a date. Your doctor can prescribe medications to help. You can use the patch, gum, or lozenges as well. You can taper off the nicotine by switching to cigarettes with lower levels prior to quitting, or join a smoking cessation group.

Most health departments offer the Cooper-Clayton Method. The social support will really help. Go online to the American Lung Association website for other resources on how to quit.

Step one is simply to make the decision and pick a date. Next, plot a plan of attack and stick to it. You can do it just like millions of others have done it before you. I wish my mom had done it. Don't wait until it's too late. Make the commitment and then follow through on it. Doing what you say you're going to do shows integrity. Don't be a shallow brook. They're noisy.

Complete the statement below: I resolve to quit smoking for myself and for my family. My method of quitting will be

________________ and I set ________________as my quit date.

Signature ________________________ Date ______________

Shallow Brooks Are Noisy

Shallow brooks are noisy with the water rushing over the rocks. The saying also applies to people. Some people talk a lot but have trouble backing up what they say—all talk and no action you might say. I always resigned myself to be the opposite, to be a person who follows-through.

When my neighbor's son-in-law from Ohio talked about hiking to the bottom of the Grand Canyon, I said I'd like to do it again one day. I did it twice when I was 20 years old. One day I got an e-mail with an invite. Their family group was planning a trip for September. They would meet at the Canyon's south rim and spend a night or two at the top. Next, they would hike seven miles of switchback trails with a one-mile vertical drop to the Canyon's bottom. The group would spend two nights at the bottom in the rustic Phantom Ranch. Lastly, they planned to hike out to the top on the easier trail, the one used by mules. At the top, they'd patch up their damaged feet and spend the night at a lodge on the rim.

I agreed to do it and recruited my wife Pia for the adventure. Once I commit, I have great follow through. I never considered myself a shallow brook and always did what I said. This was a huge and potentially painful commitment. It was common for hikers to lose toenails from the constant pounding against their hiking boots on the way down. The park rangers advised taping each toe, taping over each toe and then lubricating the tape with Vaseline. What had I gotten us into? Would my wonderful wife ever forgive me?

My healthy habits were fairly well ingrained by this point. My exercise was regular, I ate a healthy diet, and I maintained the proper weight. I simply wasn't in the habit of hiking into canyons a mile deep. I altered my training a bit to include the stair stepper machine. This was good preparation strengthening my calves, my thighs, and my knees. It was rigorous exercise, a necessary evil to survive the challenge. I continued my other cardio workouts on the elliptical, along with some strength training. All of this would serve me well.

We started at the rim trailhead before sunrise and headed down. My wife and I were with a group of veteran, annual Canyon goers who really knew the ropes, so we were in good hands. Our new friends wore lights on their heads to keep their hands free. Many of them used a walking stick in each hand. The first couple of hours, we hiked along steep cliffs in the dark winding our way down a series of switchbacks. One misstep could prove deadly. Once the sun came up we had awe-inspiring views of God's masterpiece with brilliant colors unfolding before our eyes. The Colorado River was just a thin line on the canyon floor below. Millions of years in the making, this canyon was every bit as spiritual as the grandest cathedral in the world. No doubt, God was here all around us.

About half way down was the only shade on the seven-mile trek. To enjoy it, you had to sit against the side of a composting toilet. The stench was a worthwhile trade-off for the shade. The temperature had risen to 100+ degrees. I was drinking lots of water, as was the rest of our group. It's the main thing we carried in our packs. A gallon and a half is recommended for each person. The rest of our gear went down on the backs of the mules.

A mule train of tourists was headed away from the composting toilets as we arrived. The mules come from Tennessee and go through a rigorous selection and training process before tourists ever get on their backs. A large percentage of them flunk out. Only a select few are chosen to carry people. It's a tough life going in and out of that canyon in the heat of the summer. The pack mules are the ones that didn't make the cut. They weren't calm enough to have people on them. These mules traveled in the cool of the night loaded down with precious cargo headed to Phantom Ranch, such as beer, wine, and steaks.

Five and a half hours after leaving the south rim, we were at the bottom. The temperature was around 114 degrees. There was some comfort knowing that it was a dry heat. People say this in a way that makes it almost seem pleasant, but it's hot and it feels hot. I'm pretty sure it would kill you if you didn't take care.

We checked into the ranch, took off our gear, and went and sat in the creek. When you do this, you experience relief and disbelief at the same time. It's hard to imagine water in this desert being so freezing cold. Wow, did it feel good.

Afternoons at the ranch are best spent napping in your bunkhouse or continuing to sit in the creek. It's just too hot to do much else. There is also a canteen area where you can sit and play cards while drinking cold beer. Because of heat exhaustion, the game has to be simple. Most of us had shed our hiking boots and had on camp shoes. I had blistered feet and a black toenail or two from the hike down. Surprisingly, I had fared better than I expected.

Our group spent two nights at the bottom for recovery. We ate boxed lunches provided by the ranch, and we had beef stew for dinner. I never thought beef stew could taste this good. At this point, we were refueling for the hike out. Our outbound hike would start early in the pre-dawn. The idea is to get in some distance before the heat. Getting out of the Canyon on foot is hard work. There are lots of switchbacks including the notorious section called the Devil's Corkscrew. This effort took serious determination and perseverance. Prior to my health conversion, I never would have made it.

I did remarkably well on the way back up. About midway, there was a stream where we could take off our shirts and soak them for cooling purposes, which felt great. At another point, there was the Bright Angel Campground with water available. This was a welcome rest stop prior to the final assent. We also had the luxury of those nice composting toilets there. I was in the lead group for the last few miles up. My legs were burning, but I was breathing remarkably well. The training had paid off. I was proud of myself and my level of conditioning. After all, the hike out was one vertical mile in serious heat and nine miles of switchback trails.

Finally at the top, I was overwhelmed with a sense of accomplishment. After all, this was a serious hike even for a young person. I had done it! A feeling of pride rushed upon me as I looked out over the Canyon and realized that I had conquered it.

It was a good lesson in setting goals and working towards them. The trip also helped validate the healthy habits I practice and the cardio-respiratory fitness that I maintain. This is a trip that can kill people and mules and yet at 49 years old, I came out a winner. Since then, I've hiked it one more time with my friend Mark Johnson from St. Paul Methodist Church. Talk about an inspiration. Mark conquered the canyon with two artificial hips. Mark's daily weight lifting routine and his exercise regimen made it all possible. I'm sure there was some prayer involved as well.

It all starts with determination. I was determined to set a goal, to work towards it, and to accomplish it. I made an inner commitment to get healthy enough for the challenge, which required action and preparation versus talk. I didn't talk about it much. I simply did the things I needed to do.

You can do the same. Adopt a determination to make better choices, to get healthy, and to do healthy things. Set some achievable goals first. Then set some goals that stretch you a bit more. Don't be a shallow brook. Depth of commitment plus action equals success. You can choose health for yourself and for your family. Have the courage to change and make the investment in your health, not just for now but for your future.

Exercise Intensity

There's no doubt that hiking into and out of the Grand Canyon requires a healthy heart. There's a fancy term for heart health called cardio-respiratory fitness. It means that the heart and lungs work together efficiently to carry you through life. Combined, they are the power plant for your body. If either of them gets compromised, you're in trouble. Walking is good exercise, and it's a great way to start on the road to health. Jogging and running are even better once you establish baseline fitness. The heart has to be pushed a little to stay strong.

The idea is to get to where you can exercise at 60-80 percent of your maximum heart rate. An initial goal of 50-55 percent maximum heart rate is appropriate for sedentary, out of shape individuals. This is a good start but you'll want to go higher. When you exercise at the 60 percent level, you could have a conversation, but it may take some effort. At 80 percent, it's harder to carry on a conversation. Start with the number 220 and subtract your age. This is roughly your maximum heart rate. Next, multiply your max rate by 60 percent and then by 80 percent. Ideally, this is the range you should exercise in for a healthy heart. Most exercise machines have heart rate readouts. If you're trying to jog outdoors, wear a heart rate monitor. These are fairly inexpensive.

Provided that you've just graduated from walking, make it your goal to get to the 60 percent level. An elliptical machine or a treadmill will serve the purpose. You could even be like one of the early exercise pioneers and jog outdoors. If you started your journey as a sedentary non-exerciser, shoot for cardio exercise three to four times a week. Keep an exercise journal and record when you exercised, for how long, and the level of exertion (either heart rate or rating from one to ten).

You can get these journals at a bookstore. Shoot for doing 30-40 minutes per session. Twenty minutes is OK if you're just starting out.

Thirty minutes duration most days of the week is a good goal. If you have a hard time exercising alone, try using an MP3 player and listen to music with a good beat. If that doesn't work, join an exercise group at a gym.

Try to get into a pattern of cardio exercise every other day. To start, mark it on your calendar or put it in your planner. Force yourself to stick to the pattern. It takes several weeks to establish a new habit. You'll have to force it at first. Over time, it will get easier and will become more enjoyable. You'll start to feel better and you'll be proud of yourself. Each time you exercise, you'll be strengthening your heart. Remember, fifty percent of all first time heart attack patients have one thing in common: they die. Do you really want to mess with those odds?

Your cardio fitness routine needs to be part of your lifestyle. How long will you need to do it? Forever. It's part of your job to stay healthy for later in life, for yourself, for your family, and even for your employer. Adding these exercise sessions several days a week will be one of the best things you've ever done for yourself. You will sleep better, you'll experience less stress, you'll have more energy, your breathing will improve, and you'll normalize your weight. Most importantly, your power plant will be strong and will be able to carry you through life. Moving through life without progressive and debilitating diseases is so much easier. I've seen so many disabled patients who just struggle to get through each day. Many diseases are preventable, but to prevent them, you really have to take care of your heart and maintain cardio-respiratory fitness.

4. CHANGING FROM THE INSIDE OUT
Attitude Adjustment

THERE IS A BOOK called *The Power of Positive Thinking.* Essentially, our thoughts precede our emotions and our responses to life. It all gets down to the age old question, is the glass half empty or is it half full? Do you tend to think more negatively or more positively? It truly makes a difference. It colors all of your experiences, and it affects your health.

My brother Todd is an eternal optimist. He views all problems as opportunities. When jogging, most people whine about hills. They complain, and they huff and puff. I used to run with this maniac.

"Great opportunity" he would say.

He even considers walking up long flights of steps as opportunities. When moving heavy furniture like refrigerators, washers, sleeper sofas, and huge chest freezers, brother Todd also framed these experiences as opportunities to test his muscles. He has a positive attitude, and you can develop one as well. I asked Todd to offer some thoughts on the matter, and they're listed below. Believe me; his insights will really help you.

Attitude is Everything by Todd Oetken, CFP

Early in my hotel career I was in charge of the meetings and banquets set-up crew. It was our job to place all the chairs and tables in each meeting room according to the meeting planner's specifications. I worked in a 1300 room property with over 40 meeting rooms so at times this task could be difficult. Changing a meeting room set-up from a small banquet setting for 100 to a theatre setting for 3000 could take hours. It was a job that required long physical hours to accomplish the task. However, it was a job in which I had one of those life-changing moments.

It came to me in a very subtle way, but it has stuck with me for a lifetime. It happened one April day in 1983, in a pre-convention meeting with a meeting planner of a very large convention. We were discussing all of his meeting requirements when we discovered that we had a mistake on the start and ending time of two meetings. The meeting planner informed us that he needed our ballroom turned from a banquet setting for 500 to a theater setting for 4000 within 90 minutes.

I immediately spoke up and said, "I believe my crew will have a problem delivering and setting that many chairs in that time allotment. Is there any way you could postpone the start of the second meeting by a couple of hours?"

This is where I had my life changing moment. The meeting planner looked straight at me and said, "You may be right but would you do one thing? Would you just replace the word 'problem' with the word 'challenge' and then re-state what you just said?"

I complied with his request and said, "I think it may be a challenge for my crew to turn that room over in the amount of time you requested."

Immediately my whole outlook changed and the task at hand became a challenge to me and my crew to accomplish what seemed to be impossible. My attitude went from already believing it couldn't be done to being determined to get it done in the time frame given. When I approached my staff with the task excited about this challenge, they in turn became excited, and we decided to make it happen.

When the time came, we accomplished the task with a couple of minutes to spare. What seemed to be impossibility became a competition and a morale building accomplishment, all because this man made me extricate the word "problem" from my vocabulary. I adopted this practice into my management style. In every leadership role I have had since that day in 1983 I have instructed my staff to never come to me with a problem. It was ingrained into all of my managers that they were encouraged to seek my advice or guidance on opportunities or challenges, but I would not listen to a statement, which included the word "problem." Changing the word "problem" doesn't change the severity of the task or situation but replacing it with the words "challenge" or "opportunity" changes the way your mind addresses the task. Attitude really is everything.

I have also transferred this same thought process to my personal life. I believe you should start each day by choosing to have a "grandtastic" day. I believe the way you approach your day is a choice. You cannot choose how the circumstance of each day may appear, but you can choose how you react to and deal with those circumstances.

There may be days when bad things happen. That is a fact of life. However, reacting to those bad things in a negative way does nothing to help you. I choose to find the positive in almost every negative. Each negative circumstance gives me the opportunity to grow and learn something new. It may be just pushing my tolerance of pain or increasing my confidence in dealing with adversity, but it is still my choice.

I have had colleagues who will allow other people to affect their outlook on their day or life in general. I always tell these people that only you can choose to have a bad day. You cannot choose how other people treat you but you can choose how you allow other people to affect you.

Throughout my kids' lives, I made sure that they knew that happiness and life fulfillment was their choice. I put a note in their lunch bag almost every day telling them how special they were and to choose to have a grandtastic day. This note was never even acknowledged, but as they moved out of the house I would hear them tell their friends about the notes, and I would hear my positive messages in their vocabulary. When they got to college my lunch notes were replaced with a weekly call that told them of a specific learning opportunity in my life and how they could learn from my mistakes. I would make a point of telling them how special they were to me and to the world. I would let them know that God has given them an unusual amount of positive attributes and talents, so he must really be expecting a lot out of them. Attitude is everything.

My brother Todd is so right. The attitude you choose towards life will help you in so many areas, including your health. Think positive thoughts and do positive things. Your mind represents one side of the mind, body, spirit triangle that can guide you through a healthy and successful life. Remember that the top of the triangle is a peak and with the right attitude, you can get there.

There really are no problems in life, just challenges and growth opportunities. Face them head on, and do it now. Don't put it off. If you're in the fat lane of life or even the emergency lane, you can do so much better. Step up to the starting line and run the good race. It's true that life is a marathon and you can finish strong. You just have to take that first step and have the right attitude.

Research studies show that people who are positive generally stay healthier than those who are negative. They get sick less often and bounce back quicker when they do get sick. Their immune systems are in better shape, so they're better able to cope with the bad things that come along. Attitude also proves influential in people diagnosed with chronic illness. Positive people respond better to treatment regimens, handle limitations better, and are more likely to beat their diseases than people who think the worst. As I mentioned before, my dad has had Parkinson's for 19 years and still finds opportunities everyday for personal growth.

Some people have more trouble being positive than others. They've had childhoods growing up with negative, critical parents. If you're in this category then face it. When you catch yourself being negative, write it in a journal. Also, write down the opposite way you could have thought about or responded to the situation you went through. If you're plagued by negative thoughts, wear a rubber band on your wrist and snap it each time you have one. We psychologists call this positive punishment. The technique is effective at eliminating bad habits and can work for you, too.

Keep yourself healthy by thinking positive thoughts and by expecting positive outcomes. Create an affirmation to repeat to yourself, and say it until you believe it. This is preventative medicine. For example,

"I, Chris, am a life giving spirit. I live in harmony in the here and now according to God's laws and the laws of nature. I will not accept sickness of the mind or the body." Another one I've used is "I, Chris, am happy, healthy, smart, and successful."

Write your own affirmation and use it several times a day. Tons of research validates the mind/body connection. Think positive, be positive, and act positive just for the health of it. You can do it! Make the commitment. Reflect for a moment on the message that you need to give yourself, something you need to program deep into your subconscious mind. Write it in the space below and then say it daily until you believe it. ______________________________

____

____

____

____

My Mini-Marathon Moment

When I was in my teens and twenties I was in decent shape. I ran a couple of half-marathons with various family members. They were painful of course, and I didn't break any speed records. The main thing was just to finish. I remember my time being 2:04 for the 13.2 miles. In the first few days after the race, I had intense memories of the event because I had severe pain every time I took a step. Ibuprofen was a must, and I resolved that I'd never run again.

The mini-marathon faded into distant memory as years and careers moved on. Bad habits, lack of exercise, and junk food, made another attempt highly unlikely. A mini-marathon is an effort worthy of your hunter-gatherer ancestors who ran after and tracked their meals for miles before they could eat them. As the years progressed from my thirties to my forties, the middle aged spread had taken hold. That spare tire was hard to carry a mile much less 13.2. How did people do it, I wondered? Why did they do it?

I was 49 years old when my 13-year-old daughter, Sophia, said she was going to run the race. She didn't run it, but I credit her with planting the seed in my head. I pondered the idea and it intrigued me. Could I do it at age 49? I'd have to train for it. I owned no running shoes. I hadn't run in years. Was I nuts to even consider it? The race was at the end of April, giving me about three months to prepare. What a great idea I thought. What a sense of accomplishment I would feel. I decided to try it with the goal of just finishing.

By this time, I had already established base-line fitness. I was doing my 10,000 steps a day, cardio machines 30 minutes four times a week, and I was eating a healthy high fiber/low fat diet. I would need to train for the grueling distance of 13 miles, but first I'd have to solidify the commitment. I went to a local running store, the kind where they work with you and make sure you're fitted into the right running shoes. You even have to step outside and run on the sidewalk while they watch you. It's quite a process and the clerk gives you a lot of attention. The folks at Swag's Sports Shoes in South Louisville were determined to get me into the right shoe with the proper fit.

There was some name calling, however. They called me a pronator and also diagnosed me with borderline club feet. Interestingly, this had been my nickname since I was a child (Clubfoot). These people were sharp, skillful, and intuitive. The nice lady noticed the enormous bunions on the side of my feet and just shook her head. She committed to do her best with what she had to work with. I'd need a large shoe with a wide toe box and a shoe built for stability since my ankles rolled inward with each step. I'd need to spend a good chunk of change to solidify my commitment to the race. Being very frugal by nature, I wasn't about to waste $100 and then not follow through. We found just the right thing, a New Balance Stability Shoe built for people with problem feet. I bought them and sealed the deal.

I altered my elliptical training to include intervals. First I'd do a five-minute warm up. Then, I would do three minutes at 65 RPM's. Lastly, I'd add a one-minute sprint at 80 RPMs. I would repeat this for 30 minutes. I extended this to 40 minutes at least four days a week. In the following weeks, I alternated days of intervals with days of keeping my heart rate elevated by staying at a consistent 75 RPMs. As the race drew near, I moved to the treadmill. I attempted running eight-minute miles for 30 minutes. I extended this to 45-minutes and then to one hour. I started to believe that I could actually run the race. About two weeks prior to the race, I visited the course and ran the hills in Iroquois Park that were part of the racecourse. I'd have to survive those two miles of hills as part of the 13.2-miles.

Race day is an adventure. Races start early, the weather's unpredictable, and you have to manage your urination and elimination needs along with the other 10,000 participants. Timing is important. I anxiously stood in the port-a-potty line. I was nervous. I hadn't run a race in years. Technically, I wasn't even registered because the race entries were maxed out. I was running solo, and had nobody with me. Was I nuts? Would I survive? What had I gotten myself into? I was 49 years old, a non-runner with bad feet. I needed a plan.

I spotted my salvation, a pacesetter holding up a sign with 2:00 on it. He planned to set a pace to finish in two hours. The folks clustering around him had the same goal. In my 20s I ran a 2:04. Maybe I could do it. No, I would do it, I thought. I got as close to that man as I could. I memorized his face. I focused on the sign. I visualized myself at the finish line with cheering fans on both sides. This pacesetter would pull me through; he would motivate me.

The gun sounded, and we were off. I stuck with my pacesetter and made it the first couple of miles and then through the hills. Four miles later, I was in the flats with only nine miles to go. I hung tight with my group, maybe six or eight of us. Our pace guy shouted out a joke every mile to distract us from the pain. It helped. At every water stop, I drank as much as I could without choking. Halfway through, I ate some electrolyte beans for energy. This helped as well.

At about four miles to go, I felt pretty good and moved ahead of my group. I locked onto the nice scenery ahead of me and just tried to keep up. The last mile was pure hell and it seemed like ten miles. Finally, I crossed the finish line and a rush of adrenaline surged through my body. I had done it! My time was 1:58, not bad for an old non-runner with bad feet. Just a couple of years ago, this would have been unthinkable. What an accomplishment. I was amazed with myself.

You can be amazed with yourself too. It doesn't have to be a half-marathon or climbing Mount Everest, but it's good to have a goal. Maybe it's a 5-K run, a 20-mile cycling trip, or a hike to Clingman's Dome in the Smokey Mountains. Once you start changing your lifestyle, you'll be able to do more than you think. Choose something that's doable in the future and work towards it. You'll need both short-term and long-term goals to stay motivated. Write your goal down somewhere you can see it. Buy the shoes, or book the trip. Go ahead and make the commitment.

Plan to succeed. I succeeded, and I know you will too. Making the commitment gets you halfway there so don't put it off. Setting physical, personal, professional, and other life goals is all part of constructing a balanced life. As a challenge to myself, I plan to_____________________________ in the future and set a tentative date of _________________ for accomplishing this goal.

- I plan to achieve this goal and have chosen _______________ as a witness to this commitment.
- Witness Signature ____________________________________
- Signature _______________________ Date _______________

Mad, Sad, Glad, Scared

Are you a person who wears his feelings on his sleeves or do you bottle them up and keep them corked in tight? Most of us do the second. We stuff feelings inside and let them bounce around doing all kinds of damage to our system. Lots of physical symptoms are psychosomatic and they are caused by emotional factors. These are things like rapid heart rate, stomach problems, headaches, fatigue, chest pains, and muscle aches.

In the past, kitchens came equipped with pressure cookers. These were big pots with locking lids and a steam vent on the side. The vent was meant to release steam and keep the pressure at a safe level, hence the phrase "letting off steam." If the vent was tightly closed, then excess pressure would build to the point it became dangerous. Eventually, the pot would explode, shooting the lid into the air and scalding hot water and food would fly all over the kitchen: not a pretty sight at all and very dangerous.

Your feelings are like the steam, and your mouth is your pressure release valve. The pot represents your body, which is damaged if everything is kept building up inside. Repressed feelings can cause lots and lots of problems. Some of these occur quickly, although some affect us more gradually over time. It's an important part of your health regimen to learn to let off steam by putting your feelings into words. I'm sure you can do it, and I'll tell you how.

When you're mad, sad, glad, or scared put it into words. Own the feelings rather than blaming them on somebody else. Then, talk to the person who's involved by using the formula below:

When you ______________________, I feel ____________ because ______________________________ In the future could you please

____

Initially, using the formula will be a bit uncomfortable. You'll need to force saying it to the people in your life. Believe me, it's worth the effort. Over time, it will get easier to express your feelings, and you'll feel much better as the result.

We expect people in our lives to be mind readers and to be able to figure out what we're upset about. None of us has this skill. Getting your feelings out is good for you, and you should do it sooner rather than later. Open the valve on the pressure cooker and let those feelings escape. Letting pressure build up inside puts your health at risk and in some cases it puts your relationships at risk.

Decide now that you can let go of old habits of interacting and adopt new ones. If you have unresolved anger or grudges from the past either let them go or resolve them with the person involved. Maybe you've bottled up emotions related to someone who's died. Write a letter to that person whether it's your mom, dad, brother, or anyone else. Resolve the issues and symbolically send the letter to heaven by safely burning it outside (maybe in a grill). Let go of all the emotions as the smoke rises into the sky.

Feelings are neither good nor bad. They're just part of the human condition. Talk about them. I promise it will help you in the long run. Don't be a pressure cooker. It simply won't work. When the pressure cooker blows, it makes a real mess. If something doesn't work, quit using it. If you do what you've always done, you get what you've always gotten.

Passion

Have you ever been involved in an activity where you're so engrossed and fulfilled that you lose all track of time? I can think of three things that I have encountered: hiking to the bottom of the Grand Canyon, snow skiing, and working as a missionary at a Guatemalan orphanage. I've been at the orphanage three times and am currently in the "commodore" dining room writing this chapter. In my hometown, I lose myself when I'm engaged in helping others. It's so fulfilling to me to be in a servant role and fulfilling a need for somebody else.

I have a passion for helping my 95-year-old neighbor Corinne. It totally gets me out of my own head, and gives me great joy. She thanks me all of the time and says she could never repay me, but I don't expect anything from her. You should never give expecting to receive. To give is the get. Maybe you're struggling through life without passion, enduring a job or family situation you don't like. Sometimes we have to do things out of necessity, but without passion you're sure to lose your joy.

Try to remember several times in your life when you felt totally alive, engrossed in what you were doing, totally fulfilled and joyful. List them below.

Ponder these memories one at a time. Close your eyes and picture the scene, the activities involved, the place, the colors, the smells, and the emotions. Wouldn't you like to have more of these experiences? Reflect on your current life situation, where you live, your family, your job, church, and responsibilities. Choose an area of focus, a place where you can insert passion and joy into your life. It could be work related, a hobby, volunteer work, or experiencing something with your family.

Think of yourself and imagine that you've just turned on a joy meter that goes from one to ten. Where's the joy in your life in general? Is it a three or four? Maybe it's even lower. Where would you like to be in terms of that number, maybe a seven or eight? Take some steps to get there. Joy is one of those priceless qualities that improves all aspects of your health and your life. Don't start tomorrow. Start today by signing the contract and choosing an accountability partner.

- I ____________________ commit to add joy and passion to my life by doing __________________________ on a regular basis. I will report to my accountability partner

  ____

- Signature / Date _____________________________________
- Witness / Date ______________________________________

Hurried To Death

Do you feel hurried, stressed out, and overloaded? Are you short on time and long on commitments? Does the day get away from you as you try to get everything done? What describes you the best; human being or human doing? Are you trying to do it all and not doing it at all well? You may be hurrying yourself to death.

Chronic stress is not your friend. It not only causes you to be in distress but it damages your immune system at the same time. Think of your immune system as your body guard. It constantly protects you from attacks on your body. It works 24/7. Without it you'd be sick all of the time, catch every illness that comes along, and you'd develop terminal conditions that will kill you. An AIDS patient doesn't really die from AIDS; the patient dies from the diseases the immune system would typically neutralize if it were working properly.

Let's say you were worth lots and lots of money and were doing business in a third world country. Without a body guard, you wouldn't last long. Criminal elements would be out to get you and do you harm. Knowing that your survival was at stake, would you give your bodyguard the week off? Of course not. You'd need that protection 24/7. This is what you get from your immune system, 24/7 protection. Chronic stress chips away at your defenses putting you at risk for all kinds of problems.

If you're alive you have stress. This is certainly better than the alternative. Stress has to be managed or it becomes distress. Medication can address your anxiety symptoms but the problematic lifestyle remains. You can take the battery out of a smoke detector that keeps going off but the fire will still kill you. The symptoms are trying to tell you something. Pay attention!

You may have trouble sleeping at night or experience high blood pressure and rapid heartbeat. You might find yourself easily agitated and prone to losing your cool. Maybe you grip the wheel of your car with the intensity required to squeeze all the juice out of an orange. You hurry through your day rushing between activities. Perhaps you start to wonder if you turned off the coffee maker or stove as you're driving away from home. At night you might find yourself using alcohol to take the edge off. Sometimes you burn your tongue with hot coffee or hot food because you don't have time to let it cool first. Stress can cause you to lock your keys in your car or even lock yourself out of your own house.

I hope you're not to the extremes I've described, but humor me. Think about a number between one and ten to rate your general level of stress. One is low stress with no anxiety symptoms. Five is average manageable stress with some symptoms. Ten is a distressed, driven, type A person with too much to do in too little time. If you're at a ten you can't relax and you have multiple anxiety symptoms that are not well managed. You're probably on track to have a heart attack or a stroke. Remember that 50 percent of first-time heart attack patients have one thing in common...............they die! Be honest and write your number in the following space_____. Now, could your number be lower?

Decide today that you can lower your stress level and preserve your immune system. Take some simple steps as follows:

- Don't take on more than you can do.
- Build extra time into your schedule for the unexpected.
- Allow some time gaps between commitments.
- Allow extra time for commuting. Plan to observe the speed limit.
- Take a couple of deep breaths every hour and observe the tension in your muscles at that time. This creates awareness.
- Try to do 20–30 minutes of relaxation/quiet time each day. Use a relaxation CD or nature recording if this helps. Think happy and positive thoughts.
- Laugh.
- Exercise.
- Talk things out with a friend.
- Have some fun.
- Learn to say no.
- Prepare lunches the night before.
- Make bulk meals on the weekend so you can just microwave things during your work week.
- Play.
- Take a mental health day.

Whether you're a career person, a homemaker or even a college student, everyone can take simple steps to preserve their immune system. Once it's damaged, it's hard to get back. Decide on several things you can do and write them down.

Life Balance

Once when I was in high school (pre-driving license) a friend named Greg from St. X High School convinced me to ride my bike with him 30 miles on a two-lane road to camp out with a buddy in Lebanon Junction, Kentucky. I had neither camped nor biked on a long trip before. I mistakenly packed all my gear in a green army duffle and put the straps over my shoulder.

On Saturday morning we were off biking down Preston Highway with duffle bags hanging from our sides. Each time I pedaled the duffle would pull my bike to the right, oftentimes even off the road. I had to lean left into the traffic to counteract being off balance to the right. When cars came, I erred on the side of going off into the ditch versus into the traffic. I went off into the ditch several times. It was a busy road and not really made for cyclists.

Talk about being worn out, worn down, and totally exhausted. You can be briefly off balance without too much trouble, but being off balance long term puts you at risk for all kinds of problems. The result is more than just stress—it becomes distress.

Balance involves staying centered and not getting over-weighted in one area or another. Think of the areas of your life: working, playing, relationships, spirituality, finances, health, family, and recreation. Review each area and assign it a number between one and ten based on your satisfaction. Ten means you're really satisfied, five is so-so, and one is very dissatisfied. It can also be any number in between.

- Romance / Intimacy
- Spiritual

- Family
- Friends
- Money
- Career
- Life Purpose
- Fun
- Recreation
- Health
- Physical
- Environment

Are you happy with these numbers? What might you do to improve some areas and have more balance? What would you do differently? A balanced life is one that can be sustained and one that yields the most happiness and contentment. Good balance also preserves your health, protects your immune system, and helps you live a longer more satisfying life.

If your life is way out of balance, don't freak out. You can change. Resolve to do better. Congratulations. You've just created awareness and now have a place to start.

Self-care is so important and life balance is a big part of it. If you've ever flown, you've heard the speech about putting the mask on yourself first before trying to help your children or others. Without self-care you're no good to anyone. Take care of yourself first.

Quiet Time

It's 5:30 AM and once again I'm quietly writing in an empty cafeteria in the orphanage in Guatemala City. There's something about the early quiet that refreshes, calms, restores, and renews the soul. The hustle and bustle of the city hasn't started. The gunshots outside our sanctuary walls have subsided, the prostitutes have gone home, and there's a window of quiet before the city's rush hour starts.

I use this time for quiet reflection, contemplation, and to just sit and notice my thoughts. I start by taking three deep breaths and holding them before release. Next, I notice the rhythm of my breathing. Breathing is mostly unconscious, but the rhythm repeats itself thousands of times a day. On the in-breath, I think the words "I am." On the out-breaths I hear the word "calm." I simply stay with this pattern and my mind turns inward. You can call this spiritual time, relaxation, meditation, or whatever you like. It's really the process that matters, not what you call it.

Some minutes into this the mind travels inward and you achieve what is called the relaxation response. Random thoughts drift into your consciousness. Think of them as clouds. Notice them and let them drift past. Let your mind return to relaxed emptiness receiving the next random thoughts that pass through. The process takes you deeper into a very relaxed state. Usually it will last about 20 minutes. Set your watch alarm if you're on a tight schedule, so you don't worry about running over.

Daily quiet time is a gift you need to give yourself. Remember what I said about the airplane and that oxygen mask. Self-care makes you more effective with others. God intended for you to have quiet time daily. It gets dark early for a reason. Winter was designed for more extended periods of downtime. Slow and quiet have lost their value in our busy world.

I'm not suggesting you become a slug or a slacker. I am suggesting you carve out 20 minutes of quiet time each day for yourself. Many of the things you use need to be recharged like cell phones, laptops, and shavers. If you run anything 24/7 it's going to break down. Pick a time and try this technique of quiet time for a week. After your quiet time, jot down thoughts that jumped out at you in a journal. A Higher Power may be nudging you all the time, but the quiet times might be when you're most receptive. Ponder these thoughts as you go through the day.

Quiet time has many benefits. It repairs your immune system, it can lower your blood pressure, it decreases your stress, and it gives you a calmness you can't get otherwise. Lastly, you may get in touch with divine thoughts and the leanings of your Higher Power, which can give you insights into your life and your purpose.

Try it out. Sit in a comfortable chair, but don't lie down. Place both feet on the floor. Don't cross your legs. Then, relax and start the process. Keep a journal and pen next to your chair to use afterwards. You deserve this time, and it will make you much more effective during the rest of your day. Lastly, sign the contract below.

- I commit to 20 minutes of quiet time daily for one week. My accountability partner will be ____________________________ and I will report my progress to him / her.
- Name ____
- Witness ____________________________ Date _______________

Screen Time

It's amazing how screen time has taken over the lives of most Americans. In the Guatemalan orphanage the "screen" time for the children is two hours total per week. On Sunday afternoon they watch a movie or "television." All the other time is filled easily, and they are never bored.

The kids spend time in school. They make wood-working projects, swim, play soccer, go to church, and take walks. They pray and they socialize with each other and with missionaries. They have absolutely no exposure to on-screen violence or sex. What's the result? The kids are kind, loving, respectful, happy, godly, and hard working. It's incredible to think they were raised on dumps, eating garbage, were abused and/or neglected prior to arriving at this sanctuary.

Technology is a mixed blessing. It allows you to do so much, but there's also a take-away factor. Screen time takes away from face-to-face personal relationships, time with family, face-to-face contact with friends, and can detract from social interaction skills. Also, it takes away time from physical activity. I consider screen time anything that has a monitor: cell phone, I-Phone, TV, computer monitor, or a game system. Some screen time is essential for work and school, but other screen time has the take-away factor and can also be very addictive.

Consider the amount of screen time you use. Count everything that isn't essential to your school or work. Keep a daily log in your pocket and track it for a typical day. Write the number of hours below and be honest. Total daily screen time_______________

Consider alternative activities that might be more productive, such as conversation with your significant other, exercise, helping a neighbor, volunteer work, church activities, one-on-one time with your kids, or grandkids, and so on. List them below.

Productive Alternatives

1. ____

2. ____

3. ____

4. ____

In Guatemala, the kids appreciate the two hours of screen time a week. In America, this would cause a major revolt. Think in terms of two hours a day. This includes all non-essential screen time that isn't school or work related—like Face-book, MySpace, e-mails, I-phones, game systems, TV, and Netflix. I encourage you to look at your total hours of screen time and then try to reduce it to two hours. Substitute the more productive activities you listed. You may have some initial withdrawal but this will pass. Try the two hours daily for a week. You can always relapse to your old ways.

I realize that some computer time is necessary for work and for school. There could be lengthy periods of time, such as an eight hour workday, or all evening on a computer doing college research. Try to incorporate some exercise into these periods if at all possible. There's a pedal device that sits on the floor that can go under your desk. It's possible to pedal while you're doing computer work. You could also get up every 45 minutes and walk around your office building or around the block. Return calls on your cell phone during this time. The same thing can be done in your home.

Be creative. There are even desks that adjust to standing height. Try to stand and work for a while. This burns lots more calories than sitting and lessens your chance of DVT's (blood clots) in your legs.

It's ironic that in such a poor country as Guatemala that the children look healthier than American kids. I have to think that physical activity vs. screen time has something to do with it. The problem affects adults and kids alike. Become resolved to change some of these patterns in your life. You'll be amazed at the benefits and blessings you'll receive. Sign the contract below.

I _________________________ resolve to reduce my total screen time to two hours daily for one week from _____________ to __________________ as a trial experiment. I will have my family and children do the same.

Laughter Is Good Medicine

I like watching babies because they display the whole range of emotions. Basically, they're uninhibited. At times they cry, but at other times they laugh easily. Sometimes they laugh for no apparent reason whatsoever. I've noticed this at the coffee house that I frequent. It just takes eye contact and a smile on my part for a baby to laugh. It seems to come so naturally.

School aged kids also laugh a lot. I've witnessed this at food stores and at the ice cream stores in my town. They make funny noises and laugh at themselves. Sometimes they make weird gestures. At other times they say quirky things. The important thing is that laughter is the result.

Teenage girls laugh too, but for them it's more of a cackling sound. I think they laugh at other people more than they laugh at themselves. The main thing is that even teenagers still have the capacity for spontaneous joy. They seem to be able to laugh and have fun with each other especially if they think you're not watching. Only later will they use the word "boring."

Even though laughter is good medicine, grown-ups seem to have moved away from it. Some of us have to pay a comedian to make us laugh. Oftentimes, our laughter is confined to the inside of a movie theatre. It's like scheduled laughter—laughter by appointment. God forbid that we laugh spontaneously in the course of our days. After all, we have been taught life is serious.

My youngest sister Kerri never learned the adult laughter prohibition rule. She laughs frequently and even goes out of her way to help other people laugh. Kerri is always entertaining. She entertains the food deliveryman, the mailman, and all of her neighbors. She's a prankster at heart and isn't particular about who she teases. People laugh whenever they're around her and the laughter is infectious.

If you don't have a wonderful and funny sister like Kerri, then adopt a laughter pal, someone who brings you up and not down. Hang out with someone who makes you laugh. There are grown-ups who haven't forgotten how to do it and it feels so good. Look for humor as you go through the course of your day and don't be afraid to lighten up. You'll live longer.

In Louisville, there's even a psychiatrist by the name of Cliff Kuhn, who caught the laughter bug. He calls himself "the laugh doctor." He's performed in local comedy clubs and I think he's even performed nationally. I don't know if laughter is more effective than Prozac, but the good doctor certainly thinks it helps. It's a natural way to increase the brain chemicals that help you feel happier and decrease your stress. I have to believe that it helps your immune system and makes for a longer life.

That inner child is still inside of you. Experiment with ways to tap into it even if it seems silly. There's no age limit on laughter. Seriousness might be over-rated and it might be killing you. Resolve to lighten up a bit. Pay for laughs if that helps get you started. Go to a comedy club or watch Comedy Central on TV. Rent a funny DVD or see a comedy on the big screen. Take some tips from watching children or hang out with a laughter buddy.

Having been around some people who are downright jovial, I have no doubt that laughter is good medicine. Make it part of your wellness program. Don't put it off. Life can really be serious at times.

Regular laughter needs to be one of your coping mechanisms. Good luck and good laughs!

Life's Purpose

Most of us have taken trips either for vacation or for business. We never just wander aimlessly. Generally, we know the destination and have an idea of how we'll get there. Some of us use GPS, MapQuest, or maybe even an old fashioned roadmap. Without guidance we'd be lost.

I was on a small sailboat once and having a great time. I could sight a spot on the horizon and actually sail towards it. I had good control over where I was going. Even when the wind shifted, I could make the adjustments needed to stay on course. The rudder kept the boat on course and moving in the right direction. The keel keeps the boat even (even keel).

Sometimes life can be tricky. The storms of life can toss you in every direction. When things come at you from all different sides, you need a good rudder to keep you on track. Without it you're just at the mercy of circumstances. You need a mission statement that will help guide you through life.

Mission statements are part of every company's culture these days. Large companies and small companies have them. Even fast food companies have them. At times you can see them posted on the wall inside of Wendy's, McDonald's, Taco Bell, and other large corporations. They serve as the guiding principle for the corporation. The general mission dictates the specific details of how things are done and influences how the final product is delivered.

You need your own mission statement for the same reason that big companies have them. It will help you reflect on what you're doing with your life and give you a rudder to keep you on track and traveling the right direction. If you know your mission, then decision-making gets a lot easier. Each of us makes thousands of decisions daily. A mission statement might not decrease the number of decisions, but it will help you make the right ones more often.

There's a formula I've used over the years. I've used it for so long, I truly don't remember if it's original or if I picked it up somewhere. I do know that it works for me and that it will work for you, too. You simply start out by doing some self-reflection and by filling in the blanks. Let's try it:

- I love to . . .
- I am (personality characteristics) . . . .
- I'd like to be recognized for . . . .
- My past experiences have shaped me to. . . .
- And have taught me . . . .
- My life's purpose is to (mission statement) . . . .

Your mission statement captures information from the other sections and summarizes your guiding life principle.

Having a purpose and knowing what it is gives you the rudder you need to guide you through life and also helps you to be even keel. It reduces your stress and helps contribute to your overall wellness. It helps you make decisions and lets you know which way to go. Your mission statement is your life rudder. Once you're satisfied with it, write it on an index card. Carry it in your pocket for a while until you know it by heart. When the storms of life come, you'll have the rudder you need to keep you on course. Happy sailing!

5. WELLNESS AND THE WAY FORWARD

SEVERAL YEARS AGO my niece Amy was graduating from IU with a degree in business and marketing. Amy had always been healthy and energetic, so I decided to engage her in a new venture. It started with a dinner meeting at the Texas Roadhouse in Bloomington, Indiana. I had hatched an idea for a business that would target the problem of childhood obesity and Amy would become my accomplice. We called it Fit-Kids by Catt and started it in Louisville.

Initially we researched the problem and brain-stormed solutions. Amy, my wife Pia, and I came up with a unique approach that would change the lifestyle of an entire family. We avoided identifying the overweight kid as the problem. The parents and the child would have to attend weekly education sessions on Sunday night, participate in preparing healthy food, and take part in cardio-fun-fitness activities. Niece Amy made it all fun. Families loved it!

The program ran 10 weeks with each week having a different focus: fast food, fruits, sugar, carbohydrates, and so forth. Each week the families would leave with homework to do and food logs to keep. They'd rate their progress weekly and we'd have weekly weigh-ins for all family members. Usually overweight kids have overweight parents, since acorns don't fall far from the tree. Each member of the family wore a pedometer and strived to get in 10,000 steps a day. The families really got into it. Weight loss was simply a side effect of the life-style change. The cost of teaching healthy habits for life and transforming a family's lifestyle to a healthy one was about $330 a month or roughly $1000 total.

Amy, my wife Pia, and I, ran several groups through the program. We had good success; kids lost weight, parents lost weight, and the kid's self-esteem went up. Unfortunately, we were never able to get insurance companies to place a premium on prevention. We even had parents who worked at corporate headquarters of insurance companies who couldn't get the program approved. Eventually, the good people at Baptist/Milestone Wellness took the program over and Amy continued her quest to teach families healthy lifestyles. After about a year and a half, the program was discontinued. Without insurance backing, families simply couldn't afford the monthly fee.

Preventing childhood obesity ideally should fall on parents anyway. If you have children this is your job, not mine, not my niece's, not Baptist Milestone's, and not the government's. Your overweight child or grandchild is at high risk for type II diabetes, high blood pressure, high cholesterol, and heart problems. School kids can be mean, and letting your child or grandchild become over-weight makes him or her a target for bullies. In general, overweight children grow up having less self-esteem in comparison to a child of average weight. You wouldn't knowingly let your kid eat poison and yet excess sugar, soft drinks, fried foods, and Trans fats all fall into this same category. Fast food isn't a food group and shouldn't be a staple in a child's diet.

You want your children to get good grades in school. What's their grade for healthy habits? Kids should eat five to nine fruits and vegetables a day, have three dairy products, limit their fat/sugar intake and be active for one hour each day. Is your child making the grade? Get them off the fast food habit, encourage them to try new things like fish or turkey, switch them from the burger joint to Subway, and get them away from electronic devices. Two-hours daily should be the total time in front of a monitor of any kind. This includes TV, computer, cell phone, and video games. If they have to use a video game, make it an active one like a Wii sports system. Encourage walking, biking, and going to the park. In some neighborhoods it's safe enough for kids in a group to walk to school. You might even walk with them.

In the words of childhood obesity and wellness expert Amy Oetken, "Teach your kids healthy habits that will last a lifetime." There are lots of resources out there that can show you how. Step up to the plate as a parent and have your kids push the plate away if it's the wrong stuff. Don't saddle your children with health problems that are totally preventable. If you're a grandparent, maybe you could be influential as well.

You can do it and you should start today. Go to the USDA website as a resource to get started. If you Google childhood obesity on the web, you'll find links to all kinds of helpful resources. Even the President's wife, Michelle Obama, has jumped on the bandwagon and is helping bring attention to this pressing problem in America.

Baseline Fitness

Being physically fit at age 51 is a very good thing. My prevention program and my health maintenance have kept me in very good shape. I'm probably in better shape than 95 percent of most people my age. Today I'm entering the final day of my Guatemalan mission trip at the Hogar Rafael Ayau Orphanage. It's about 6 AM and I'm sitting in the dining room once again reflecting on my time. The experience has been both physical and spiritual. I'm totally recharged, just like when you click the battery icon on your laptop and see the 100 % readout.

My healthy lifestyle has served me well. By day, I've cut grass, weeded gardens, trimmed some trees, and other physical activities. Dinner is a welcome respite from the physical activity. Immediately after dinner comes more physical activity. The older girls have gym time. They want to play both soccer and full court basketball. It takes even more endurance than the day work. I'm the oldest missionary of the group. Two others on the missionary team are in their 30s and one in his 20s. In spite of my age, I'm able to endure one and a half to two hours sprinting back and forth across the gym. Guatemala City is a mile high, the same elevation as Denver. It takes extra endurance at this altitude.

Latin American soccer is serious stuff. The teenage girls are fast, aggressive, and can dribble the ball right around me. I sprinted non-stop, yelled at the top of my lungs, had the time of my life, yet touched the ball only a small percentage of the time. I took one really hard fall and split my elbow open when a girl undercut me. I have thin blood since I take an 81 mg aspirin each day, so the amount of blood made the injury look worse than it really was. I injured my knee and ripped my pants when I hit the floor in a hard slide trying to stop a goal. Also I banged my head on the floor after colliding with one of the teenagers.

After returning to my room I immediately took 800 mg of Ibuprofen. Sure I was a little banged up, but each day in Guatemala I was able to work hard and play hard all day and all evening long. I had the time of my life. Prevention and health maintenance make all the difference in the quality of your life. It makes a difference both now and in the future.

Project yourself down the road towards your retirement years. Whether you retire at 55, 65, or 70, don't you want to have your health left to do the things that are important to you, fill you with passion, and give you great joy? Why spend your golden years going to doctors, taking boatloads of medicines, having surgeries, and not being mobile. Health in retirement is like a US Savings Bond: you can invest now for the future payoff. In this case you get an immediate pay off as well. I'm thrilled to know that my investments are paying off. My health is great. I feel great. I can travel and I have mobility. My mind works well, and I can use all of this to help others. Invest more in yourself and invest regularly. It's like the concept of dollar-cost-averaging with the stock market. You start early, invest regular amounts at regular intervals, and you have money reserves as your work-life winds down.

The slow, steady, and consistent tortoise wins the race. The hare runs at full speed, doesn't rest, and can't finish the race set out before him, and I have to think the hare gets high blood pressure, diabetes, peripheral artery disease, emphysema, osteoporosis, heart disease, Alzheimer's, and a whole litany of other problems.

Choose to be the tortoise, steady and deliberate. Your trip towards the finish will be much healthier.

COMING HOME

I'm writing this final section on the plane coming home from Guatemala. My week of mission work in the orphanage was great, but at some point we all have to come home. The nice thing about travel is that it opens your eyes, gives you some reference points, and in some cases reveals sharp contrasts in cultures. I experienced all of these on my most recent trip.

In Guatemala, you see some fast food joints, but trips to these seem more like a luxury rather than part of daily life. In general, it seems that Guatemalan people are of a shorter stature than Americans. If they ate like Americans, they would all look obese. This is far from the case. I'm not sure which food pyramid they follow, but for the most part, they eat fruits, vegetables, beans, tortillas, and maybe some chicken, fish or pork. Sweets and high fat junk foods are not usually part of the diet. Obesity doesn't seem to be a big issue.

The contrast in cultures is really evident at the airport. Guatemala City has a newly built, modern airport. It has shops, a nice restaurant, modern gates, Wi-Fi, and a duty free area. It doesn't have electric carts that drive people who can't walk fast enough to their gates as they do in the USA. There really doesn't seem to be a need for them. If there's an overweight person in the airport, it's a rare occurrence, and the person is typically an American.

Coming home is hard, especially during the transition process. You have to get past several gatekeepers. I went through security first and was patted down twice. My carry-on-bag was searched at the gate, and I was patted down a third time. I even had a question or two to verify that the passport was truly mine. If I ever had the guts to assume another's identity, I wouldn't choose a middle aged balding psychologist and would become someone like George Clooney or Brad Pitt instead.

LEAVING LIFE IN THE FAT LANE

Usually, once on the plane and seated, my anxiety goes down. Not this time. My wife had booked me in the exit row due to my 6’4” frame and my disdain for having my knees scrunched up in my face. The exit row usually gives me a good feeling. This time was different. Across the aisle from me was an obese American man also in an exit row. The stewardess was going through the exit row lecture to make sure everyone was comfortable performing the exit row duties “in the rare event of an emergency.” I had an uneasy feeling.

In the middle of the exit row lecture, the man interrupted the stewardess. She was in the middle of asking if everyone was fit to perform the duties. At that point, the overweight American had the bad judgment and the bad timing to ask if he could have a seat belt extension. He was frustrated and was doing everything in his power to cram his large belly in behind the seat belt. This man was struggling, and we were nowhere close to an emergency yet. He seemed winded as well. The stewardess had to explain the obvious by saying, “You can’t wear seatbelt extensions in an exit row.” Upon hearing the bad news, the man became more determined than ever and eventually made the buckle click. He was in no shape to help himself much less anyone else.

Coming home from Central America typically involves a stop in Houston, Atlanta, or Miami. My transfer was in Atlanta, but the sights are the same at all three places. The most striking thing is the amount of obesity you see immediately upon touching down in the USA. Obese people can’t move fast enough to get to their gates on time, so oftentimes, the attendants who drive the electric carts have to assist them. They drive the carts between gates, push wheelchairs, and load and unload these people for the airlines as priority passengers. Technically, they're disabled because they've lost their health and their activities of daily living have become impaired. It's a contrast that really hits home when you return from a country where people only eat as much as they need without all the excess. Usually, excess is not an option.

There's an immediate awareness of the differences in the diets as well. At the Atlanta airport there are hundreds of restaurants: fast food, slow food, moo goo food, etc. I'm a curious person, so I always try to see what people are eating. You can do this from the hallway without actually stepping into an airport restaurant. I surveyed several places and couldn't help but notice cheeseburgers and fries, buffalo chicken wings, biscuits and gravy, and salads, but only with thick, artery clogging creamy dressings, like bleu cheese, ranch, or Thousand Island. I did see something like a Fresh Express, but the line there was minimal.

Coming home is really a rude awakening. It's an awakening to the terrible things we as Americans are doing to our bodies. Our unhealthy diets and our unhealthy lifestyles create a burden, not just for us, but also for society as a whole. Our collective habits keep driving up the cost of healthcare and driving down life expectancy and our quality of life. When a third of all American kids are obese, what do you think that says about our future? Obesity is an epidemic that is creating a drain on our economy that will be passed onto the next generation. It helps sustain the disease model of medicine, creating problems like heart disease, diabetes, sleep apnea, degenerative joints, and strokes.

Ideally, we need to turn the corner and adopt a new mindset. It starts with you and the changes you've made as part of reading this book. It spreads when you teach healthy lifestyle habits to your children, your grandchildren, or pass on some information to a friend. The changes need to then move from the individual to the culture.

At this point, the average life expectancy of Americans is going backwards. You can't change society but you can do your part to make changes yourself and be a positive role model for your family and for other people you know. Start by getting your own health in order and then reach a bit further by spreading the word. We really need a culture that rewards wellness rather than disease. It really can start with you. Resolve to make the changes you learned about in this book and tell someone you're going to do it. Sign the change contract if that helps. Don't put it off and don't start and stop. A lifestyle is a style that suits you for life. Preserving the quality of life starts with you. Don't delay. This is your chance. This is your moment. Just do it!

Who Pays the Piper

Whatever happened to the concept of personal responsibility? I own a car, and I take care of it. Periodically, I rotate the tires, change the oil, change other fluids, and get it tuned up. I am totally responsible for the upkeep and the expense if it breaks down. If you have a car, you operate with this same mentality.

What makes healthcare different? Why do people destroy their health and then expect insurance companies or the government to pay for it? The logic is really flawed and doesn't apply to any other thing we have or use. I practice prevention, pay out-of-pocket for what minimal health care costs I have, and I don't expect anyone else to own my problems. Resolve yourself to be in control of your health. Don't get into the victim mentality.

Prevention and personal responsibility are the answers to the health care debate. Rewards should be attached to prevention through a variety of incentives. These could come through tax rebates, decreased insurance premiums, reduced Medicare taxes, and so forth. I have to believe that an ounce of prevention costs less than a pound of cure.

Health and prevention should become a priority for everyone in the U.S. There isn't any health care plan that can replace personal responsibility and accountability. There truly needs to be a giant shift in thinking about health. Sweeping change can't happen all at once, but a small part of it can start with you. There truly needs to be a shift from the disease model to the wellness model. The right choices today will put you in control of your health and wellness both now and in the future.

Adopt the practices I've advocated in this book. If you have kids or grandkids, teach them what you learned. They'll be able to adopt a healthy lifestyle sooner rather than later. Today's kids are already predicted to have a shorter lifespan than their parents and for the first time in history, the lifespan of Americans in general, has gone backwards.

Conclusion and Well Wishes

In closing this book, I wish you well on your journey through life. With perseverance you can improve both your health and your habits. You can be healthier, happier, more productive, and feel better overall. The quality of your life can improve and you can preserve your health for the future by practicing wellness. The fact that you've read this far means you're ready to change.

If you haven't already done it, get started today. Start at square one. Make the first change then build on it. Enlist your accountability partner, someone who will keep you honest. Map out your journey and follow the route. Get out or stay out of the fat lane of life. Wellness and prevention will keep you on course. Let your gradual changes become a lifestyle. Little by little, you'll develop healthy habits that will last a lifetime. With health on your side, your life journey will be so much better.

As you go on from here I wish you well, and most of all, I wish you wellness.

-Dr. Chris Catt, PSYD, HSPP, ACSM

APPENDIX

DISCUSSION QUESTIONS for STUDENTS

1. Discuss the trans-theoretical model of change and how it parallels Dr. Catt's experience. Address the pre-contemplation, contemplation, preparation, action, and the maintenance phases.
2. Evaluate the environmental, social, occupational, spiritual, physical, intellectual, and emotional components of wellness as these apply to Dr. Catt's lifestyle prior to his wellness conversion. On a 1-10 scale, also rate how you're doing in each of these areas.
3. At some point Dr. Catt had self-efficacy, which enabled him to achieve his goals. Discuss the importance of this concept. Next, think about times in your life when you experienced an outcome that was either positively or negatively influenced by your thoughts about the goal. Share these with your class.
4. Todd Oetken writes a section in the book about attitude. What is it about attitude that links it so strongly to behavior change? Are there any areas in your life where you could use an attitude adjustment? Talk this over in your discussion group.
5. Equate the following with each of the five stages of change: I won't, I may, I will, I am, I am still. How is knowing a person's stage of readiness to change so important in helping him/her with the change process?
6. What challenges did Dr. Catt face as he contemplated changing his habits and which ones were ongoing as he progressed through the wellness process? What challenges do you face as

you consider making a positive behavior change? Discuss these.

7. Consider Dr. Catt's analogy of the body being a vehicle. How do you treat a vehicle to get the most miles out of it and keep it in good running condition? Project yourself twenty years older, when most bodies start breaking down. Speculate on what you might do along the way to minimize health problems and keep your body running strong.
8. Differentiate internal versus external locus of control. Apply the concept to Dr. Catt's experience and its relationship to his success or failure. How would you categorize your own locus of control? Talk about it with your discussion group. If possible, give examples.
9. How is wellness a process rather than a goal? Discuss the pros and cons of looking at wellness in each of these ways. Which viewpoint would be most beneficial in the long run?
10. Dr. Catt was successful in changing his ways. Past success usually feeds future success. Describe the best experience you ever had setting a goal, working towards it, and achieving it. Share this with the group.
11. What similarities are there between Dr. Catt's unhealthy habits and some that you may see in your parents? It's human nature to repeat what we know. How do you plan to avoid repeating unhealthy habits you've witnessed within your family?
12. Discuss the lifestyle diseases Dr. Catt had and brainstorm preventative activities that will help keep you from traveling down the same road.

13. Specifically identify something you need to change regarding your health and habits. Using the trans-theoretical model, evaluate your readiness to change. If you're at the right stage, make the commitment and enlist an accountability partner.

www.ingramcontent.com/pod-product-compliance
Lightning Source LLC
LaVergne TN
LVHW020626100826
845148LV00012B/2070

9781583742488